D0871776

STEREOTYPED MOVEMENTS

STEREOTYPED MOVEMENTS

Brain and Behavior Relationships

Robert L. Sprague
Karl M. Newell
Editors

AMERICAN PSYCHOLOGICAL ASSOCIATION

WASHINGTON, DC

Published by
American Psychological Association
750 First Street, NE
Washington, DC 20002

Copies may be ordered from
APA Order Department
P.O. Box 2710
Hyattsville, MD 20784

In the UK and Europe, copies may be ordered from
American Psychological Association
3 Henrietta Street
Covent Garden, London
WC2E 8LU England

Typeset in Minion by University Graphics, Inc., York, PA
Printer: Princeton Academic Press, Inc., Lawrenceville, NJ
Cover Designer: Rohani Design, Edmonds, WA. Illustration © Michael Rohani, 1996.
Technical/Production Editor: Sarah J. Trembath

Library of Congress Cataloging-in-Publication Data
Stereotyped movements : brain and behavior relationships / edited by
  Robert L. Sprague and Karl M. Newell.
      p.   cm.
  Includes bibliographical references and indexes.
  ISBN 1-55798-301-1
  1. Stereotyped behavior (Psychiatry) I. Sprague, Robert L.
  II. Newell, Karl M., 1945–   .
  RC569.5.S74S74   1996   96-4732
  616.8—dc20   CIP

British Library Cataloguing-in-Publication Data
A CIP record is available from the British Library

Printed in the United States of America
First edition

APA Science Volumes

The Suggestibility of Children's Recollections: Implications for Eyewitness Testimony

Taste, Experience, and Feeding: Development and Learning

Temperament: Individual Differences at the Interface of Biology and Behavior

Through the Looking Glass: Issues of Psychological Well-Being in Captive Nonhuman Primates

APA expects to publish volumes on the following conference topics:

Attribution Processes, Person Perception, and Social Interaction: The Legacy of Ned Jones

Changing Ecological Approaches to Development: Organism–Environment Mutualities

Children Exposed to Family Violence

Conceptual Structure and Processes: Emergence, Discovery, and Change

Genetic, Ethological, and Evolutionary Perspectives on Human Development

Global Prospects for Education: Development, Culture, and Schooling

Maintaining and Promoting Integrity in Behavioral Science Research

Marital and Family Therapy Outcome and Process Research

Measuring Changes in Patients Following Psychological and Pharmacological Interventions

Psychology Beyond the Threshold: Conference on General and Applied Experimental Psychology and a Festschrift for William N. Dember

Psychology of Industrial Relations

Psychophysiological Study of Attention

As part of its continuing and expanding commitment to enhance the dissemination of scientific psychological knowledge, the Science Directorate of the APA established a Scientific Conferences Program. A series of volumes resulting from these conferences is produced jointly by the Science Directorate and the Office of Communications. A call for proposals is issued twice annually by the Scientific Directorate, which, collaboratively with the APA Board of Scientific Affairs, evaluates the proposals and selects several conferences for funding. This important effort has resulted in an exceptional series of meetings and scholarly volumes, each of which has contributed to the dissemination of research and dialogue in these topical areas.

The APA Science Directorate's conferences funding program has supported 40 conferences since its inception in 1988. To date, 28 volumes resulting from conferences have been published.

WILLIAM C. HOWELL, PHD
Executive Director

VIRGINIA E. HOLT
Assistant Executive Director

Contents

Contributors

Alan J. Beauchamp, Northern Michigan University
Gershon Berkson, University of Illinois at Chicago
James W. Bodfish, Western Carolina Center, Morgantown, North Carolina
Daniel E. Casey, VA Medical Center, Portland, Oregon
Margaret P. Creedon, Human-Michael Reese Hospital, Chicago, Illinois
Joshua Fryman, University of Florida
John P. Gluck, University of New Mexico
Mark H. Lewis, University of Florida
Richard B. Mailman, University of North Carolina
Ralph G. Maurer, University of Florida Medical School
Karl M. Newell, Pennsylvania State University
Jaun R. Sanchez-Ramos, School of Medicine, University of Miami
Lisa M. Shulman, School of Medicine, University of Miami, Florida
Robert L. Sprague, University of Illinois
Osnat B. Teitelbaum, University of Florida
Philip Teitelbaum, University of Florida
Esther Thelen, Indiana University
Joel Vilensky, Indiana University School of Medicine
William J. Weiner, School of Medicine, University of Miami, Florida

Preface

Children raised in institutionalized environments often develop aimless, repetitive movements known as *stereotypies*. Because these stereotyped movements are so obviously different than the movement patterns of normal children, they have attracted clinical and research interest for a number of years. When one begins to examine the phenomenon, one becomes aware that there are obvious parallels in animal behavior, particularly the stereotyped pacing of caged animals. About 40 years ago, with the advent of psychoactive medication to treat psychiatric patients and mentally retarded individuals, it became obvious that long-term use of neuroleptic medication also produced stereotyped movements, which were labeled *tardive dyskinesia.*

We have individually conducted research for a number of years and subsequently worked together the past 9 years on some aspects of stereotypy, particularly tardive dyskinesia. However, when faced with the various proposed causes of stereotyped movements, we began to see a need to gather together the knowledge of researchers working on various aspects of stereotyped movements. The field of stereotyped movements has been disjointed: One group of researchers is interested in the tardive dyskinetic movements of psychiatric patients treated with neuroleptics; another group is interested in the stereotyped mannerisms of developmentally disabled institutionalized children; and still another group is interested in following the developmental path of such behavior in normal children, which may appear for a brief period of time then disappear with maturation. Typically each of these groups has its own set of assumptions and methodologies, and has no overarching theory to tie all of these aspects together. Such divergence poses considerable problems for the advance of knowledge. Thus, the question was raised as to how the editors could best address the situation by attempting to review the state of affairs and making a contribution to the advancement of knowledge.

Because it was apparent that none of the diverse groups had an overall perspective, we decided to bring together in one volume the work and reflections of these diverse researchers. We hope that this collection will mark a beginning of researchers' efforts to bring synthesis to the field of stereotyped movements and help point the way to further study.

From the beginning, we realized that researchers from different disciplines and with different research interests should be included. It was obvious that some investigators with a human developmental point of view should be involved, as well as those with perspectives informed by the use of animal subjects. Because a number of movement disorders are primarily caused by biomedical disorders, we decided to include biomedical researchers. It was also obvious that if any thorough understanding of the multiply determined, complex stereotypes is to be reached, input must be obtained from both basic research laboratories and clinics that deal with practical problems of patients showing symptoms of various disorders.

The Science Directorate of the American Psychological Association gave a firm commitment to the plan for the execution of these ideas. Additional support was obtained from the Department of Kinesiology and the Institute for Research on Human Development of the University of Illinois. After considerable work, and with more delays than expected, this book is the culmination of these efforts. It is hoped that *Stereotyped Movements: Brain and Behavior Relationships* will be helpful in pointing toward new directions in this area.

Introduction

Robert L. Sprague and Karl M. Newell

Repetitive movements, termed *stereotypy*, have become the focus of attention of a number of researchers working with children and adults with developmental disabilities and clinicians who work in residential facilities for these individuals. Although a number of articles about stereotypies have been written and published in various sources—including animal, psychiatric, psychological, and medical publications—there are very few comprehensive books on the topic. This book is an attempt to fill the need for an integrated examination of and commentary on stereotyped movements.

CONCEPT OF STEREOTYPY

The concept of repetitive motions without purpose is about 300 years old. In 1701 Nehemia Grew wrote, "We see also Mad people . . . run upon some one action . . . without variation" (Frith & Done, 1990, p. 232). Since that early recognition of aimless repetition of movements in a clinical population, the concept of stereotypy has, until recent years, been used primarily in the clinical literature. However, even though the importance of stereotyped actions has been widely acknowledged in the clinical literature, the theoretical and empirical coverage of the topic has been sparse and uneven. For example, Frith and Done (1990) pointed out that a well-known handbook in psychiatry mentions the importance of stereotyped behavior in its introduction and then never mentions the topic again. Such an uneven treatment of the topic of stereotypy is not unusual. Even in this day of computerized databases and even though stereotypy has been studied for years, the term *stereotypy* is not a descriptor in the widely used PsycINFO database. It is not surprising, then, that there is not a coherent conceptual and empirical understanding of the importance of stereotyped behavior in the literature at this time.

DEFINING STEREOTYPY

It is usually necessary to have a conceptual framework and commonly accepted definition of a concept before an area of behavioral investigation can fully or creatively develop. In the absence of a commonly accepted definition an area of study often flounders. This appears to be the case with the concept of stereotyped behavior. Although a number of books have discussed stereotyped behavior, the definition of stereotypy varies considerably. This is particularly true of the books that have recently appeared linking stereotypy with the more general topic of movement disorders (Lang & Weiner, 1992; Shah & Donald, 1986; Weiner & Lang, 1989).

In one of the few books that extensively covers the topic of stereotypy from the biological perspective—*Neurobiology of Stereotyped Behaviour* (Cooper & Dourish, 1990b)—the behaviors mentioned in the definition of stereotypy are varied and extensive. The introductory chapter to Cooper and Dourish's book offers no definition for what the chapters to follow contain (Cooper & Dourish, 1990a). Near the end of Cooper and Dourish's book, however, Frith and Done (1990) point out the difficulties of defining stereotypy by mentioning the domains of the behavior that need to be considered: (a) complexity, (b) coordination, and (c) degree of conscious control. Frith and Done also list the terms used to indicate repetitive behavior in the wide range of behavioral domains in which stereotypy is a problem: (a) tremor, (b) tics, (c) tardive dyskinesia, (4) perseveration, (e) mannerisms, and (f) obsessions. Thus, rather than narrowing the concept down to a reasonable, understandable level, the authors probably broaden the potential phenomenological domain by cogently pointing out the difficulties with current definitions.

Stossel (1990) defines stereotypy as "repetitive, purposeless, and involuntary, often interfering with normal behaviour" (p. 260). In a more extensive explanation of stereotypy Stossel introduces the dimensions of excess activity, hyperkinesis, and decreased activity (hypokinesis) as important domains in defining the behavior. Such elaborations do not clarify, but rather, make the meaning of stereotypy more vague when the concept of hypokinesis is included.

The most comprehensive inclusive list of repetitive behaviors for clinical conditions is given by Lohr and Wisniewski (1987). They list types of repetitive behaviors that occur in the following wide range of clinical symptomatology: frontal lobe damage, dementia, schizophrenia, postencephalitic states, catatonia, autism, congenital deafness, congenital blindness, mental retardation, agitated depression, and obsessive–compulsive disorders, as well as Tourette's syndrome, psychomotor epilepsy, psychogenic fugue states, alcoholic blackouts, twilight state of unknown origin, Asperger's syndrome, and a few other diseases. Thus, there is little doubt from Lohr and Wisniewski's list of clinical disorders that stereotypy is a pervasive symptom that deserves adequate research attention.

Differential diagnosis is a major problem with such a broad range of diseases. In an attempt to improve the ability to diagnosis such a broad range of conditions, Lohr and Wisniewski (1987) present a table in which they speculate on the positive severity of the symptoms along a range of behavioral domains. Lohr and Wisniewski's criteria for stereotypy include the following: level of consciousness—high; degree of repetitiveness—high; frequency of the behavior—high; control over the motor act—very little; outward appearance of the motor act—normal or bizarre; time span of each act—short; relationship to other motor activity—little or none; purposefulness—absent; and accompaniment other diseases—frequent

(p. 92). Thus, as can be readily appreciated, repetitive motor activity is quite prevalent throughout psychopathological conditions, and accurate differential diagnosis is very difficult. The differential diagnosis of this complex condition is often not given adequate consideration in many books that address stereotypy.

For this book, the following working definition is adopted: Stereotypy is frequent repetition of a movement sequence that appears to the observer to be invariant in form and without any obvious purpose. Whether a movement sequence can be classified as stereotypy depends on the context in which it occurs. Movements similar to stereotyped movements may not be classified as stereotyped if they have some obvious purpose. For example, rocking back and forth while sitting in a chair is often categorized as stereotypy. However, if a person performed the exact same movement sequence while holding a crying baby, the movement would be interpreted as having a purpose of pacifying the baby. It should be quite apparent, however, that the observer often has difficulty in determining whether or not the movement sequence has a purpose. In these situations, the repetitive movement is likely to be classified as stereotyped if the person repeatedly engages in the movement in a variety of environmental situations, again, without any obvious purpose connecting the situations.

SUBJECTS IN STUDIES OF STEREOTYPY

There have been several contexts and population groups emphasized in the study of stereotypies. The most prevalent have been the examination of animal stereotypies and those evident in clinical human populations. Stereotypies are also present, however, in normal infant motor behavior.

Animal Studies

Most people are familiar with cage stereotypies because they were often quite apparent when one visited the older zoos, which tended to house animals, such as lions, in confined cages. Such an environment usually produced stereotypic pacing of the animals for considerable portions of the day. Research on stereotypies in animals typically is not driven by an interest in the naturalistic behavior of the animals, but, rather, by an interest in the neurobiological variables thought to be involved in the etiology of stereotyped behavior in human populations (Ellison & See, 1991; See Sant, & Ellison, 1987).

Clinical Populations

Clinical populations have been popular subjects for stereotypy researchers for a simple reason: The abnormal repetitive movements of some clinical populations are so obvious that it is difficult to ignore them. When viewing such populations as autistic children or severely mentally retarded children in care and treatment facilities, visitors often ask, "Why do these people behave in such a strange fashion as they do?" It is not easy to present a satisfactory answer as to why a person would stand in a corner rocking back and forth for considerable portions of the day without any obvious external motivator or reward for such behavior. Of course, even more puzzling to the visitor is why some of the people with stereotypic behavior engage in self-destructive acts. Although this is not a book on self-destructive behavior (SIB), there is no sharp demarcation line between stereotypy and SIB because excessive repetitive movements often blend into SIB.

Most of the research on clinical populations, however, has been with severely mentally retarded people. Psychiatric patients are often administered psychotropic medications, particularly neuroleptic medications, to control their psychotic disorders. Although such medications have been most helpful in treating psychiatric diseases, the side effect of *tardive dyskinesia*—an abnormal involuntary movement disorder often displayed in facial stereotyped movements—has been a perplexing problem. The increased significance of the problem in these populations is indicated by the large number of articles in the literature written about tardive dyskinesia (American Psychiatric Association, 1979, 1992; Fann, Smith, Davis, & Domino, 1980; Jeste & Wyatt, 1982; Wolf & Mosnaim, 1988). Thus, another line of research has developed in the general area of stereotyped movements by those researchers primarily interested in tardive dyskinesia, and includes theory and experimentation on the neurotransmitter systems involved, brain structures damaged, and the kinds of symptoms displayed.

MEASURES OF STEREOTYPY

In any area of complex behavior a number of different measurement techniques often are developed to produce empirical evidence about the phenomenon under investigation. This certainly is the case in the area of stereotypy. As in other areas of behavioral investigation, different measurement techniques tend to create separate groups of investigators who become familiar with and use only some of the methods available. Most of the human work, and much of the animal research for that matter, has used categorical observational techniques to record over time the presence and frequency of certain repetitive acts. Some of the more frequently used observational measures are rating scales, checklists, frequency counts, and global impressions. Obviously, all of these observational methods are based on a human observer watching some experimental subject and recording from memory the observations on some record form.

Although such observation techniques are quite useful, particularly at the beginning stages of a line of research, there are a number of limitations that have encouraged some researchers (e.g., Lohr & Caligiuri, 1992; May, 1987; Sprague & Newell, 1987) to employ other measurement technologies. Some of the limitations are (a) reduced accuracy in observing and recording high-speed behavior such as tremor, (b) errors introduced by relying on the observer's memory and ability to integrate the amount of stereotyped behavior over some finite period of time, (c) limitations in the ability to observe several different stereotyped movements occurring at the same time, and (d) limitations in the ability to note the antecedents in the environment and record the stereotyped behavior at the same time. Some clear-cut examples of these limitations can be cited. Physiological tremor of the finger occurs in the range of 8–10 Hz and is well beyond the limit of the human observer to detect and record accurately by natural observation, yet tremor seems to be an important indicator in many of the movement disorders.

NEED FOR INTEGRATION

To even a casual student of stereotypy it is apparent that there are different camps of researchers who usually do not communicate with each other and usually maintain separate lines of research. For instance, although some of the animal researchers are motivated by problems arising in human clinical populations, many are not. Thus, there tends to be a major division along the lines of what subjects are used in the experiments.

Another division in this area is the contrast between basic research and research driven by clinical considerations. As is true in several areas of science, the basic researchers tend not to communicate with clinicians primarily interested in solving problems associated with clinical populations. The type of measures and procedures used also tends to separate investigators into several distinct interest groups. Observation techniques, primarily rating scales and checklists, usually are employed to measure stereotyped behavior but more recently, small groups of researchers have begun to use *nonlinear dynamic measures*, which are relatively unfamiliar to most other researchers in the stereotypy area. Nonlinear dynamic measures often involve taking samplings in 2 or 3 dimensional space from several limbs of the body over periods of time typically at high rates like 100 to 200 Hz.

There are other divisions in the area of stereotypies that could be listed, but enough distinctions have been pointed out to show the fractionated nature of the mixed group of researchers currently working in stereotypy. The fractionation is promoted by, of course, the complex nature of the disorders being studied, the lack of common definitions of content, the lack of an acceptable theoretical framework, and the divergent backgrounds of the investigators. Since the problem of repetitive movements is so significant in many human populations, it seems quite obvious that more rapid progress could be made in this area if there was more communality of definitions, techniques, and theories rather than such fractionation and divergency that now seems to be the status quo. This book explores some of the divergent lines and, hopefully, will contribute to bringing some common ground to the area of stereotypy.

ORGANIZATION OF THIS BOOK

This book is divided into three parts. Part 1 covers the issue of defining stereotypy, which, as just described, is a complex issue. Part 2 attempts to understand the multiple causes of stereotyped behavior. Finally, Part 3 presents a wide range of methods for measuring stereotyped behavior, from rating-scale techniques, to dynamic systems approaches, to applied clinical measures.

Part One: Defining the Behavior

Berkson (chapter 1) begins by discussing the history of the concept of stereotypy and pointing out several important aspects of the history that reflect the traditional controversy of nature and nurture, which Berkson terms *experience* and *organismic factors* instead. Moving to the issues in the area, Berkson discusses long-term maintenance. People are usually puzzled by the long-term continuation of stereotyped behavior, which often persists without any obvious external reinforcement. The author proposes the idea of *sensory feedback* as an explanation for stereotypy resistance to extinction. He then deals with abnormal focused affections, which are less distinctive and dramatic but, nevertheless, are observable because of their compulsive and obsessive characteristics. Because stereotypy is much more commonly observed in children and adults with development delays, Berkson also explores the developmental aspect of stereotypy.

In chapter 2, Shulman, Sanchez-Ramos, and Weiner approach the problem of defining stereotypy by examining clinical disorders. This is a useful approach because it is closely tied to practical applications derived from our understanding of the disorder (Part 2), and a field is often enriched with the knowledge gained from pathological conditions. The authors briefly describe the origins of stereotypy by pointing out that these behaviors are often observed in normal infants, a topic that Thelen explains in more detail in chapter 7. There are at least three prevalent disorders in which stereotypy is often noted: autism, mental retardation, and schizophrenia. Shulman et al. briefly describe these three disorders and associated stereotypies. In the last section of the chapter they describe three other disorders that more recently have been associated with stereotypic movements: Rett syndrome, Tourette syndrome, and tardive dyskinesia, the measurement of which is further described by Sprague in chapter 5.

Part Two: Understanding the Causes

In chapter 3, which is primarily devoted to the neurobiology of stereotypy, Lewis, Gluck, Bodfish, Beauchamp, and Mailman selectively review the extensive literature in this area and describe several of their studies. From the perspective of the neuropharmacology of stereotypy, the authors review the extensive support for the hypothesis of the link between dopamine and stereotyped behavior. They cite evidence for alterations in dopamine receptor density being linked to the expression of stereotyped behavior. Much support for the dopamine involvement in stereotypy has been obtained in animal subjects. Lewis and colleagues discuss a very interesting model of early social deprivation in monkeys and its effects on developing behavior, particularly stereotypy. Clinical populations, as noted previously, often provide valuable information to supplement animal studies. The authors review stereotypy in populations of mentally retarded people and discuss blink-rate as an index of dopamine activity in this clinical population. Often, stereotypy is associated with other disorders; the authors glean important information from studies of the comorbidity of stereotypies and other disorders.

Chapter 4 by Casey discusses the effects of neuroleptic medications, which are commonly used with psychiatric patients, on tongue protrusions of monkey subjects. Abnormal, stereotyped tongue and mouth movements are commonly observed in patients exposed to neuroleptic medications who develop tardive dyskinesia (further discussed in chapter 5). Casey describes research in which both dopamine and serotonin agonists were administered to monkeys. After a period of time, the monkeys developed significantly increased tongue protrusions, which is a possible model for tardive dyskinesia in human patients.

Part Three: Measuring the Movements

Sprague (chapter 5) reviews the literature on behavioral instruments that have been developed to assess stereotyped movements in human populations. He points out that much of this literature lacks a psychometric sophistication, although it emphasizes pressing clinical problems. However, such an approach often leads to unreliable data on the prevalence and severity of the clinical symptoms, as the author indicates in the review of the studies assessing tardive dyskinesia. He argues for a change in emphasis in clinical assessment using psychometric principles proposed as standards by the American Psychological Association and other organizations interested in behavioral assessment.

Newell (chapter 6) brings new dynamic concepts and new measuring techniques to the study of stereotypy. Given the usual definitions of stereotypy, it typically is thought that the repetitive movements are highly stable and do not vary much from act to act. The author proposes that biological motion can be cast into categories of *absolute* (precise quantities of motion) and *relative* (a unique set of motion properties of the torso and limbs) movement. From this perspective, he examines the *kinematics* (measurements in time and space) of stereotyped behavior and finds that there is considerable absolute variability in the kinematics of acts perceived as stereotypic. Then he compares developmentally normal subjects who are requested to simulate a stereotyped behavior with clinical subjects who have stereotyped behavior. The kinematic variability of the stereotyped acts of the clinical subjects is greater than that of the simulated acts. Thus, the defining nature of stereotypy is questioned. Newell addresses this issue at length. The dynamic perspective of chapter 6 helps set the stage for the subsequent chapter by Thelen.

In chapter 7, Thelen writes about normal infant stereotypies. Normal infants develop repetitive rhythmical behaviors that change with the developmental age of the infant. There have been several theories proposed to explain the developmental changes in infant stereotyped behaviors, many of which are based on biological assumptions of stages of development. Using a dynamic perspective, Thelen interprets the changing infant stereotyped behavior as natural oscillations that become entrained by *attractors*, a quantitative concept indicating stability in a complex system. This is, of course, quite a different theoretical approach than stage theories. Using this perspective, she further examines the development of purposeful kicking and reaching behavior in infants.

In the last chapter (chapter 8), Teitelbaum, Maurer, Fryman, Teitelbaum, Vilensky, and Creedon begin with a discussion of experimentally lesioned animals that become *frozen*, or unable to move to one side or the other when caught in a corner. There are clinical analogs of this immobility that the authors explore at some length. It is often the case that in advanced stage of Parkinson's disease patients find it difficult to initiate walking. Extrapolating from data and concepts obtained from the animal literature, the authors fruitfully explore methods of improving the immobility states of patients.

In summary, this book begins with a history of stereotypy, reviews animal and clinical studies, considers measuring stereotypy with a variety of methods, and ends with a discussion of stereotypy in normal infants and clinical populations. Finally, the book presents evidence that dynamic approaches may be quite fruitful to integrate this theoretically diverse area and bring more complete understanding and more rapid advancements.

REFERENCES

American Psychiatric Association. (1979). *Tardive dyskinesia task force report 18.* Washington, DC: Author.

American Psychiatric Association. (1992). *Tardive dyskinesia: A task force report of the American Psychiatric Association.* Washington, DC: Author.

Cooper, S. J., & Dourish, C. T. (1990a). An introduction to the concept of stereotypy and a historical perspective on the role of brain dopamine. In S. J. Cooper and C. T. Dourish (Eds.), *Neurobiology of stereotyped behavior* (p. 1–24). New York: Oxford University Press.

Cooper, S. J., & Dourish, C. T. (Eds). (1990b). *Neurobiology of stereotyped behavior.* New York: Oxford University Press.

Ellison, G., & See, R. (1991). A computerized methodology for the study of neuroleptic-induced oral dyskinesias. In A. Boulton, G. Baker, M. Martin-Iverson
(Eds.), *Neuromethods (Vol. 18). Animal models in psychiatry.* Clifton, NJ: Human Press.

Fann, W. E., Smith, R. C., Davis, J. M., & Domino, E. F. (1980). *Tardive dyskinesia.*
New York: Sp Medical and Scientific Books.

Frith, C. D., & Done, D. J. (1990). Stereotyped behaviour in madness and in health.
In S. J. Cooper and C. T. Dourish (Eds.), *Neurobiology of stereotyped behaviour*
(p. 232–259). New York: Oxford University Press.

Jeste, D. V., & Wyatt, R. J. (1982). *Understanding and treating tardive dyskinesia.* New
York: Guilford.

Lang, A. E., & Weiner, W. J. (Eds.). (1992). *Drug-induced movement disorders.* Mt.
Kisco, NY: Futura.

Lohr, J. B., & Caligiuri, M. P. (1992). Quantitative instrumental measurement of tardive dyskinesia: A review. *Neuropsychopharmacology, 6,* 231–239.

Lohr, J. B., & Wisniewski, A. A. (1987). *Movement disorders: A neuropsychiatric approach.* New York: Guilford.

May, P. R. A. (1987). Measurement of extrapyramidal symptoms and involuntary
movements by electronic instruments. *Psychopharmacology Bulletin, 23,* 187–
188.

See, R. E., Sant, W. W., & Ellison, G. (1987). Recording oral activity in rats reveals a
long-lasting subsensitivity to haloperidol as a function of duration of previous
haloperidol treatment. *Pharmacology Biochemistry & Behavior, 28,* 175–178.

Shah, N., & Donald, A. G. (1986). *Movement disorders.* New York: Plenum.

Sprague, R. L., & Newell, K. M. (1987). Toward a movement control perspective of
tardive dyskinesia. In H. Meltzer (Ed.), *Psychopharmacology: The third generation of progress* (pp. 1233–1238). New York: Raven.

Stossel, A. J. (1990). Stereotyped motor phenomena in neurological disease. In S. J.
Cooper and C. T. Dourish (Eds.), *Neurobiology of stereotyped behavior* (pp. 260–
292). New York: Oxford University Press.

Weiner, W. J., & Lang, A. E. (1989). *Movement disorders: A comprehensive survey.*
Mount Kisco, NY: Futura.

Wolf, M. E., & Mosnaim, A. D. (Eds.). (1988). *Tardive dyskinesia: Biological mechanisms and clinical aspects.* Washington, DC. American Psychiatric Press.

PART ONE

Defining the Behavior

1

Feedback and Control in the Development of Abnormal Stereotyped Behaviors

Gershon Berkson

The term *stereotyped* has been applied to many types of behavior, including normal animal behaviors, abnormal repetitive behaviors of caged animals, body rocking and thumb sucking of socially deprived higher primates, normal repetitive behaviors of infancy, consequences of injecting high doses of stimulant drugs, dyskinesias following psychotropic drug administration, and autistic behaviors of children and adults with developmental disabilities.

Other phenomena may also be related to the general behavior class characterized by its stereotyped nature. Obsessions and compulsions, normal rigidities of childhood, clothes and food fetishes, abnormally focused affections (AFAs) are all behaviors that seem to have important factors in common with abnormal stereotyped behaviors (Bender & Schilder, 1940; Schultz & Berkson, 1995). Even normal behaviors such as those involved in the playing of video games are of a stereotyped nature.

The research reported in this chapter was supported in part by a grant from the National Institute of Child Health and Human Development (HD-27184). Laura Gutermuth, Grace Baranek, Carol Bline, Warren Phillips, and Leon Miller contributed items to the checklist described in this chapter.

Certainly, one must make important distinctions. Some stereotyped behaviors are characteristic of all members of a species, whereas some are abnormal. Some behaviors are developmentally normative; others are not. Some stereotyped behaviors are adaptive; some are not. Although some are voluntary, some are not under the person's control. In some, the motor action is evident, whereas in others, what stands out are their cognitive aspects. In some, we need to focus on the organization of an action, and in others, it is the sensory feedback that seems most important for behavioral control.

It is not yet clear whether stereotyped behaviors are best approached as parts of one large behavioral class that share a common origin and mechanism or as relatively independent phenomena with different histories and manifestations. Nor is it clear how these behaviors are developed or why they are maintained for years. That is, it is not clear why people and animals engage in stereotyped behaviors. This chapter presents a brief historical review of stereotyped behaviors and then focuses on two central questions: (a) what is the relationship among various stereotyped behaviors and (b) how are such behaviors developed and maintained.

HISTORICAL REVIEW

The study of stereotyped behaviors began seriously in the 1940s. Bender and Schilder (1940) described behaviors that are characterized by highly focused positive attention to certain ideas or activities. They differentiated these "impulsions" from obsessions and compulsions (Tuke, 1894) because impulsions are associated with positive affect, whereas obsessions are characterized by negative affect. Bender and Schilder did suggest, however, that the impulsions might be related to the primitive motor stereotypes of infancy, and that they could develop into obsessions and compulsions during adolescence. In 1944, Levy published a study that focused on the development of tics and "habits" that seemed to result from movement restraint in animals and children. Lourie (1949) speculated that the feedback from rhythmic behaviors in infancy facilitates normal motor development and cognitive growth. He believed that this feedback can come to maintain motor stereotypes such as body rocking. The ideas in these classic papers have influenced work on stereotyped behaviors during the last 50 years.

Environmental Factors

Abnormal stereotyped behaviors can be increased or reduced through alterations of the environment. Carnivores develop pacing and tic stereotyped behaviors when they are caged. Higher primates who are reared in social isolation develop body rocking and thumb sucking. Human babies engage in normal infant stereotypes, especially those who have minimal social interaction. Children who are reared in institution-like environments tend to engage in abnormal stereotyped behaviors (see Guess & Carr, 1991; Mason, 1991, 1993, for recent reviews).

Modifying the environment appropriately reduces the level of abnormal stereotyped behaviors. Mason and Berkson (1975) reported that rhesus monkey babies reared away from their natural mothers on stationary surrogate mothers develop body rocking, but that monkey babies reared on moving surrogate mothers do not. It has also been reported that normal social interaction—for even short periods—dramatically reduces the level of stereotyped behaviors in institutionalized infants who are profoundly retarded (Gallagher & Berkson, 1986). In general, studies have found that it is relatively easy to reduce the expression of stereotyped behaviors by providing alternative activities (see Thompson & Thelen, 1986, for a review and an exception).

Organismic Factors

Although enriching an individual's environment reduces abnormal stereotyped behaviors easily, such a change does not necessarily eliminate them. Organismic factors, such as the presence of visual handicap, early childhood autism, and severe mental retardation are clear predictors of the likelihood of abnormal stereotyped behaviors. This suggests that experiential factors alone are not sufficient causes. Organismic factors, working during development, probably mediate the effects of environment. In other words, a full understanding of abnormal stereotyped behaviors will come from a consideration of developmental factors (Lewis, Baumeister, & Mailman, 1987).

LONG-TERM MAINTENANCE OF STEREOTYPED BEHAVIORS

In looking at developmental factors, three levels of analysis must be considered: (a) What determines the moment-to-moment changes in the expression of stereotyped behaviors? (b) What influences bring stereotyped behaviors about in the first place? (c) What maintains the stereotyped behaviors in the behavior repertoire?

Moment-to-moment changes are determined by what else the person is doing, and by the level of general arousal, perhaps affected by certain drugs. Abnormal stereotyped behaviors probably arise from intrinsic motor patterns that are part of normal motor and cognitive development. This development of rhythmic motor patterns is what Lourie (1949; see also Thelen, 1979) emphasized as the normal starting point of abnormal stereotyped behaviors.

However, it is the third level of description, the long-term maintenance of abnormal stereotyped behaviors, that is one focus of this chapter. What are the factors that determine the dramatic maintenance of abnormal stereotyped behaviors in the behavior repertoire of persons who are blind, autistic, and severely retarded even when other aspects of their behavior (e.g., locomotion) develop normally? Another question is why a person would spend most of his or her day engaged in behaviors that have no apparent function (Baumeister, 1978).

An answer to this latter question may be that these behaviors are, in fact, adaptive. Such behaviors seem to result in a reward that comes from controlling the feedback from stereotyped behaviors. In other words, long-term maintenance of specific abnormal stereotyped behaviors may be dependent on two separate reinforcing factors. First, a specific sensory feedback associated with the behaviors seems to contribute to the maintenance of stereotyped behavior (Lovaas, Newsom, & Hickman, 1987), and second, the reinforcement that comes from control of that feedback provides

6

an independent source of maintaining the behavior (Berkson, Baranek, & Thompson, 1992; Buyer, Berkson, Winnega, & Morton, 1987; also see Emerson & Howard, 1992; Wieseler, Hanson, Chamberlain, & Thompson, 1988 for another, perhaps related, possibility).

Thus, development of abnormal stereotyped behaviors may begin with the normal stereotyped behaviors of infancy, but they are maintained, at least sometimes, for long periods of time after infancy by the reward associated with control of specific feedback (Thelen, 1981).

There is a practical problem in testing the concept that the control of sensory feedback maintains stereotyped behaviors. Sometimes feedback from certain behaviors is difficult to describe adequately. For instance, in stereotyped body rocking, it is difficult to be more precise than the idea that some kinesthetic–vestibular stimulation is important. One can exclude auditory and visual input as factors (Stewart, 1985), so a complex of kinesthetic and vestibular feedback has ordinarily been implicated by exclusion. However, attempts to test the role of kinesthetic and vestibular stimulation directly have been crude at best, and such studies have not yet separated vestibular and kinesthetic aspects of the feedback.

Perhaps the best solution to the general problem of analyzing the rewarding aspects of sensory stimulation has been to shift attention from motor stereotypes to object stereotypes and abnormal focused affections (Lovaas et al., 1987). It is simple to modify the stimulus properties of the objects that are used in a stereotyped manner (e.g., string that is "twiddled" by an autistic child). This quickly reduces the level of expression of that stereotyped behavior, at least temporarily (Lovaas et al., 1987; Winnega & Berkson, 1986).

Therefore, it is possible to identify feedback from certain stereotyped patterns; by modifying the feedback, one can effect dramatic reduction in the stereotyped behavior. This also demonstrates that feedback is important for maintaining the behavior. If feedback is important, then it seems useful to identify the kinds of stereotyped stimuli that all children enjoy controlling. In the preschool period, children may require endless routines before they can be put to bed. Some children may have clothing and food fetishes, and some play almost endlessly at video games. Older children have an almost unbelievable motivation to work at computers.

In addition to feedback, control of the feedback sometimes can be independently rewarding. In one study (Buyer et al., 1987), individuals who engaged in body rocking were provided with an opportunity to choose among three rocking chairs. The first chair was modified so that it did not rock. The second chair was rocked at the person's preferred rocking rate by another person. The third choice was a rocking chair that the subject could control. The results were clear. Individuals chose the chair that could be rocked for them over the stationary chair. However, they most often chose the rocking chair that they could control themselves. This effect was strongest in individuals with higher tested developmental levels. The Buyer et al. study was repeated in principle by Berkson, Baranek, and Thompson (1992). In the latter case, feedback from stereotyped behaviors was either under the individual's control or independent of his or her action; the control variable was demonstrated in some, but not all, cases. Thus, control of feedback from the stereotyped behaviors appears to be a factor that works in some, but not all, individuals.

RELATIONSHIP BETWEEN STEREOTYPED BEHAVIORS

The interests of some children are highly focused. For instance, one girl we worked with organized her life around the letter "S." Some individuals can always be found in the same part of the house they live in; others use highly specific and stereotyped routes of travel. Also familiar are the rare cases of savants—individuals with mental retardation or autism who have the ability to do calendar math calculations or who are skilled in the arts. These individuals all engage in behaviors that are stereotyped.

As Bender and Schilder (1940) observed, behaviors like these are highly focused and are associated with positive affect. These characteristics are referred to as AFAs; Bender and Schilder called these characteristics impulsions. AFAs may be related to the focused affections of normal hobbies, to motor stereotypes in abnormal and normal populations, and perhaps even to the rigidities, compulsions, and obsessions seen in early childhood autism and in obsessive–compulsive disorder. Underlying them all might be focused and definable feedback and the control of that feedback.

Bender and Schilder (1940) apparently believed that there was a general connection among all kinds of stereotypy, including motor stereotypes, rituals, AFAs, obsessions and compulsions, and even normal hobbies. However, they also believed that this factor was manifested differently at different ages.

In her thesis, Schultz (1992) tested the relationship between various stereotyped behaviors by using formal observations in the classroom and teacher reports of the existence of various stereotyped behaviors, including AFAs. Her study indicated that only a minimal relationship existed between observations and teacher reports. Even when specific behaviors were combined into supercategories, the agreement rate did not exceed 33% (Schultz, 1992; Schultz & Berkson, 1995).

It is not difficult to find reasons for lack of agreement between measures. Probably the most important is that the teachers' estimate (which, in this case, was confirmed by two other teachers or by one of us) summarized experience over a long time in several contexts, whereas the observations were limited in time and situation.

Beginning with the proposition that general classes of stereotyped behaviors might be related to each other, Schultz chose groups of children who either did or did not demonstrate AFAs. She then asked whether the two groups differed in their levels of other stereotyped behaviors, such as body-rocking. The simple answer was that no difference existed between the groups. That is, she found no support for an association between AFAs and motor stereotypes.

Our first attempt to look for a common factor in stereotyped and related behaviors found no such relationship. Our next attempt to look for a common factor in stereotyped and related behaviors involved the design and administration of a checklist (Gutermuth, 1993) that tapped various stereotyped behaviors. The checklist contains items that are intended to tap AFAs, conventional object and motor stereotyped behaviors, rigidities, obsessive–compulsive disorder behaviors, savant skills, and sensory defensiveness.

We first screened children who attended schools for developmentally disabled people, adults who worked in a sheltered workshop, and adults who lived in a state-operated residential program. We asked two staff members who knew these individuals well to indicate which of them engaged in stereotyped behaviors. We did this in such a way that we were not yet aware of the identities of the potential participants. We then requested consent for participation from parents and guardians of those potential participants identified as having some stereotyped behaviors.

After receiving consent, we asked two other staff people who knew the participants at least moderately well independently to complete the checklist. After this preliminary set of procedures, we emerged with data on 246 participants (i.e., we had two checklists for each participant).

An analysis of the principal components revealed evidence of a weak general stereotypy factor, the presence of which was hardly manifest. Several orthogonal factors emerged, including ones that we named *orientation to sounds or words, visual orientation, maintenance of sameness* or *rigidity, motor stereotypy,* and *object stereotypy* (Berkson, Gutermuth, & Baranek, 1995).

This study showed only weak evidence for a general stereotypy factor. There did, however, appear to be domains of stereotyped behaviors that summarized the relationships among several specific behavior patterns. In a third study, Baranek and Berkson (1994) correlated three measures of tactile defensiveness with these same orthogonal factors and showed that there seemed to be a special relationship between tactile defensiveness and the rigidity factor.

In general, these studies found little evidence for an overarching general stereotypy factor. However, these studies did indicate definable domains of stereotyped and related behaviors.

DEVELOPMENTAL CORRELATES

Although little evidence for a general factor of stereotyped behavior has been fact, the use of the word *stereotyped* encourages one to think that a general factor might exist (Aman, Richmond, Stewart, Bell, & Kissel, 1987). On the other hand, Bender and Schilder suggested that there could be a general factor that is manifested differently at different times during development. In other words, it might be better to conceive of the term *stereotyped* as denoting a loosely connected set of behaviors that have different developmental histories. Demonstrating such a proposition would require careful longitudinal studies over a significant portion of the developmental period. No such longitudinal studies have been conducted, but some cross-sectional studies exist that may be relevant to a beginning analysis. Overall, these cross-sectional studies suggest that developmental age (DA) and experiential history, rather than chronological age (CA), may be the most relevant mediating variables.

The most obvious measure to investigate is, however, CA. In children without disabilities, there seems to be a decline of stereotyped behaviors with CA. However, stereotyped movements increase with CA in individuals who are severely retarded and who live in institutional settings (Berkson, McQuiston, Jacobson, Eyman, & Borthwick, 1985). In an attempt to understand this apparent contradiction, several studies have been conducted in which CA has been separated from DA.

Among individuals with severe retardation, CA is relatively independent of DA with the correlation varying around .35. That is, the mental growth level of persons who are severely retarded is slow, although their physical growth usually parallels that of persons without disabilities. This allows researchers to separate chronological from developmental age statistically (Thompson & Berkson, 1985). Thompson and Berkson found that at least certain stereotyped behaviors exhibited by children who lived in an institutional setting were positively correlated with CA. There was a negative correlation of these stereotyped behaviors with DA.

This finding did not hold true, however, in a work by Schultz (1992) that focused on children with disabilities who lived at home and attended a well-organized school that had a stimulating educational program. In Schultz's study, as well as in Gutermuth (1993), the expected negative correlation between stereotyped behaviors and DA did occur, and the association with CA was not significant. Thus, in stimulating environments, there is a decline of stereotyped behaviors with DA. In custodial environments, as well as situations of maternal deprivation (and perhaps in case, where organismic factors prevent normal experiences), however, stereo-typed behaviors may increase. Thus, as was shown in the early animal studies reviewed (e.g., Mason & Berkson, 1975), the early environment seems to be important to whether stereotyped behaviors increase or decrease with age. However, there is always a general decline associated with DA.

These relationships with development seem to apply most to behaviors associated with infancy (e.g., body rocking). In this chapter, other behaviors (e.g., object stereotypes and AFAs) have also been included, although they require further analysis. In a preliminary study in which the interest was to define the developmental maturity of various stereotyped patterns, Gutermuth (1993) developed a method for rating the age equivalent level of various stereotyped behaviors. She did this by first categorizing most of the items on the checklist into several categories, including object stereotypes, motor stereotypes, insistence on consistency, nonword vocalizations, abnormal attachment to objects, preferred location, ritualistic behaviors, and word and phrase vocalizations. Gutermuth established the age equivalence of the categories by calculating the DA of children who demonstrated the various categories of stereotypy. She discovered that there were DA equivalents to the various stereotyped behaviors and that the age levels of the various behaviors differed significantly. For example, object and motor stereotypes tended to be associated with less maturity than AFA categories.

CONCLUSION

This chapter began with the suggestion that there may be a general factor underlying all stereotyped behaviors. The research referred to here is inconsistent with such a view. There is little evidence that there is a general tendency for a person to be stereotyped in his or her behavior (see, however, Rojahn, 1986).

This is even true of the behaviors called AFA. The behavior of some children is based on unusually focused motivational systems. However, again, at this time, the idea is only hypothetical that these motivational systems generally represent a broader tendency to be motivationally focused.

Although there is little evidence for a general stereotypy behavior class, it appears that domains of stereotyped behaviors exist (but see Rojahn, 1986). These may include domains for visual orientation, auditory and verbal orientation, rigidity or maintenance of sameness, object stereotypes, and motor stereotypes.

There also is some evidence that stereotyped behaviors are associated with developmental factors. The nature of the child's experience affects the development of stereotyped behaviors. In general, stereotyped behaviors decline with DA and are unrelated to CA, unless the child is exposed to experientially depriving environments (in which case there is a positive association of stereotyped behaviors with CA). On the other hand, certain stereotyped behaviors reflect more maturity than do others. For example, it seems as though motor stereotypes and AFAs represent different levels of adaptive behavior.

Lourie's (1949) view that the feedback from stereotyped behaviors is important in their maintenance has been supported and elaborated over the years. It appears that specific stimulation is necessary for stereotyped behaviors to be definable in some cases. It also seems as though the control of that stimulation can itself be independently rewarding. Improving the description of feedback and determining when control is or is not important are both tasks for the future.

REFERENCES

Aman, M. G., Richmond, G., Stewart, A. W., Bell, J. C., & Kissel, R. C. (1987). The Aberrant Behavior Checklist: Factor structure and the effect of subject variables in American and New Zealand facilities. *American Journal of Mental Deficiency, 91*, 570–578.

Baranek, G., & Berkson, G. (1994). *Tactile defensiveness and stereotypes: Are they related?* Paper presented at the Gatlinburg Conference on Research and Theory in Mental Retardation and Developmental Disabilities, Gatlinburg, TN.

Baumeister, A. A. (1978). Origins and control of stereotyped movements. In C. E. Meyers (Ed.), Quality of life in severely and profoundly retarded people: Research foundations for improvement (pp. 353–384). *Monograph of the American Association on Mental Deficiency, No. 3.*

Bender, L., & Schilder, P. (1940). Impulsions: A specific disorder of the behavior of children. *Archives of Neurology & Psychiatry, 44*, 990–1008.

Berkson, G., Baranek, G., & Thompson, T. (1992). *Personal control of abnormal stereotyped behaviors.* Paper presented at the Gatlinburg Conference on Research and Theory in Mental Retardation and Developmental Disabilities, Gatlinburg, TN.

Berkson, G., Gutermuth, L., & Baranek, G. (1995). Relative prevalence and relation among stereotyped and similar behaviors. *American Journal of Mental Deficiency, 100,* 137–145.

Berkson, G., McQuiston, S., Jacobson, J. W., Eyman, R., & Borthwick, S. (1985) The relationship between age and stereotyped behaviors. *Mental Retardation, 23,* 31–33.

Buyer, L. S., Berkson, G., Winnega, M., & Morton, L. (1987). Stimulation and control as components of stereotyped body-rocking. *American Journal of Mental Deficiency, 91,* 543–547.

Emerson, E., & Howard, D. (1992). Schedule-induced stereotypy. *Research in Developmental Disabilities, 13,* 335–361.

Gallagher, R. J., & Berkson, G. (1986). Effect of intervention techniques in reducing stereotypic hand gazing in young severely disabled children. *American Journal of Mental Deficiency, 91,* 170–177.

Guess, D., & Carr, E. (1991). Emergence and maintenance of stereotypy and self-injury. *American Journal of Mental Retardation, 96,* 299–319.

Gutermuth, L. E. (1993). *Developmentally related differences in stereotypical behaviors of children with developmental disabilities.* Unpublished master's thesis, University of Illinois at Chicago.

Levy, D. M. (1944). On the problem of movement restraint. *American Journal of Orthopsychiatry, 14,* 644–671.

Lewis, M. H., Baumeister, A. A., & Mailman, R. B. (1987). A neurobiological alternative to the perceptual reinforcement hypothesis of stereotyped behavior: A commentary on "Self-stimulatory behavior and perceptual reinforcement." *Journal of Applied Behavior Analysis, 20,* 253–258.

Lourie, R. S. (1949). The role of rhythmic patterns in childhood. *American Journal of Psychiatry, 105,* 653–660.

Lovaas, I., Newsom, C., & Hickman, C. (1987). Self-stimulatory behavior and perceptual reinforcement. *Journal of Applied Behavior Analysis, 20,* 45–68.

Mason, G. J. (1991). Stereotypies: A critical review. *Animal Behaviour, 41,* 1015–1037.

Mason, G. J. (1993). Forms of stereotypic behaviour. In A. B. Lawrence & J. Rushen

(Eds.), *Stereotypic animal behaviour: Fundamentals and applications to welfare* (pp. 7–40). Wallinford, England: CAB International.

Mason, W. A., & Berkson, G. (1975). Effects of maternal mobility on the development of rocking and other behaviors in rhesus monkeys: A study with artificial mothers. *Developmental Psychobiology, 8,* 197–211.

Rojahn, J. (1986). Self-injurious and stereotypic behavior of noninstitutionalized mentally retarded people: Prevalence and classification. *American Journal of Mental Deficiency, 91,* 268–276.

Schultz, T. M. (1992). *Abnormal focused affections.* Unpublished master's thesis, University of Illinois at Chicago.

Schultz, T., & Berkson, G. (1995). Definition of abnormal focused affections and exploration of their relation to abnormal stereotyped behaviors. *American Journal of Mental Retardation, 100,* 376–390.

Stewart, J. D. (1985). *Sound intensity and stereotypic body rocking in severely profoundly retarded children: A sensory reinforcement approach.* Unpublished doctoral dissertation, University of Illinois at Chicago.

Thelen, E. (1979). Rhythmical stereotypies in normal human infants. *Animal Behaviour, 27,* 699–715.

Thelen, E. (1981). Rhythmical behavior in infancy: An ethological perspective. *Developmental Psychobiology, 17,* 237–257.

Thompson, D. F., & Thelen, E. (1986). The effects of supplemental vestibular stimulation on stereotyped behavior and development in normal infants. *Physical & Occupational Therapy in Pediatrics, 6,* 57–66.

Thompson, T. J., & Berkson, G. (1985). Stereotyped behavior of severely disabled children in classroom and free-play settings. *American Journal of Mental Deficiency, 6,* 580–586.

Tuke, D. H. (1894). Imperative ideas. *Brain, 17,* 179–197.

Wieseler, N. A., Hanson, R. H., Chamberlain, T. P., & Thompson, T. (1988). Stereotypic behavior of mentally retarded adults adjunctive to a positive reinforcement schedule. *Research in Developmental Disabilities, 9,* 393–403.

Winnega, M., & Berkson, G. (1986). Analyzing the stimulus properties of objects used in stereotyped behavior. *American Journal of Mental Deficiency, 91,* 277–285.

2

Defining Features, Clinical Conditions, and Theoretical Constructs of Stereotyped Movements

Lisa M. Shulman, Juan R. Sanchez-Ramos, and
William J. Weiner

S tereotyped behavior is a difficult concept to define. This difficulty is not dissimilar to that faced in the accurate diagnosis of other movement disorders. Identification and classification can be hindered by a number of obstacles. In contrast to a paralysis of motor function or an incoordination of movement, the "material evidence" of a movement disorder is ephemeral and fleeting, occurring with variable frequency and characterized by morphologic variability. Some movement disorders are stimulus sensitive, activated by vocalization or motor activity. Most are exacerbated by emotional stress. In addition, the presence of movement disorders in the setting of psychiatric disease (e.g., schizophrenia, autism) combined with the existence of psychogenic movement disorders adds to the complexity of accurate diagnosis.

The characteristics of a given movement disorder may not be unique to a specific disease process. For example, the chorea of Huntington's disease may not appear strikingly different from the chorea that occurs as a drug-induced side effect. Therefore, a given movement disorder may cross

This work was supported in part by a grant from the National Parkinson Foundation, Miami, Florida.

the lines of neurologic, psychiatric, developmental, toxic-metabolic, hereditary, and even infectious disorders. The recognition and identification of a specific movement abnormality does not necessarily imply a specific etiologic diagnosis. The scarcity of identifiable anatomical substrates that correlate with each different movement disorder also thwart attempts at orderly categorization. The frequent usage of hybrid terms such as "choreodystonic" or "choreoathetoid" in the description of movement disorders bears testimony to the ambiguities facing the clinician who seeks to categorize abnormal movements.

The literature on stereotyped behaviors reverberates with a similar lack of clarity of definition and echoes a similar uncertainty of classification and terminology.

In this chapter, the defining features of stereotypies are explored, and the clinical conditions in which such features have been observed are reviewed. The theoretical constructs that may explain the expression of stereotypies are also presented.

TOWARD A DEFINITION OF STEREOTYPY

Certain behaviors have been labelled as stereotypies (see Table 1). Yet, what are the fundamental defining features of stereotypies? It is safest to say stereotyped behavior is identified by its repetitive quality, but precisely how stereotyped do these repetitive actions need to be? Newell, Van Emmerik, and Sprague (1992) found that low variability is not a defining feature of stereotypies associated with tardive dyskinesia. The tardive dyskinetic movements of individuals exposed to neuroleptic agents were no less variable than the simulated movements produced by healthy persons. Therefore, these repetitive movements illustrate a loss of randomness and a reduced variability, but invariability is not required.

Rhythmicity is often included in definitions of stereotypy, although it is not an essential attribute. Many common stereotypies, such as body rocking, head banging or bruxism are performed in a rhythmical manner, and rhythmic vocalizations may occur in tardive dyskinesia. However, other stereotypies are intermittent and irregular in frequency, such as the

Table 1

Common Stereotypies

Area of Body	Stereotypy
Mouth	Bruxism, lip movements, biting, grimacing, smiling, frowning, vocalizations (e.g., snorting, blowing, groaning, hissing, singing, screaming)
Head	Banging, nodding, shaking, weaving, bizarre posturing
Arms and Hands	Finger waving and flicking before the eyes, holding hand at arm's length and watching the fingers move, finger drumming or pill-rolling movements, hand rubbing, fist pounding, hand to face, mouth, or ear movements, touching or stroking parts of the body, fragments of common actions (e.g., smoking, combing hair)
Trunk	Body rocking, twirling, and circling, pelvic swaying and thrusting, sitting and arising
Legs	Jumping, hopping, lotus position, walking in circles or back and forth
Self-Injurious Behavior	Lip manipulation, hand biting, eye poking and gouging, scratching, self-beating

Note. From Kurlan, R., & O'Brien, C., Spontaneous movement disorders in psychiatric patients. In A. E. Lang & W. J. Weiner (Eds.), *Drug-induced movement disorders* (p. 261). Mt. Kisco, New York: Futura. Reprinted with permission.

posturing behavior seen in persons with schizophrenia and the eye blinking associated with Tourette's syndrome (a disorder characterized by multiple motor and vocal tics). The abrupt, transient, nonrhythmic nature of some movements may prompt researchers to label them as tics, but they are no less stereotypic in character.

Stereotypic motor behaviors appear to be extraneous, serving no obvious purpose and providing no particular benefit, although the movements may be sufficiently distracting and preoccupying to impair function. Studies of persons with profound mental retardation have suggested that controlling or eliminating stereotypy enhances learning (Koegel &

Covert, 1972). The impairment of attention in persons with Tourette's syndrome was found to correlate with the frequency of observable tics (Silverstein, Como, Palumbo, West, & Kurlan, 1992). The absence of an obvious purpose does not rule out the possibility that the stereotypies may serve a covert function for the organism.

The presence of stereotyped behaviors in persons who are congenitally blind or deaf, as well as their appearance in animals who are housed in unstimulating environments underlies the belief that stereotypies may serve a compensatory function. Recurring sequences of motor activity may be providing the stimulation that is missing from the environment. In this paradigm, the self-stimulating nature of stereotypies is considered the key component in the initiation and maintenance of these motor behaviors (Berkson & Gallagher, 1986).

Alternatively, stereotypies may be interpreted as arising in states of increased stress and thereby serving a de-arousal function. In this model, stereotyped behaviors enable the organism to dissipate frustration or anxiety with the environmental situation. Studies of the behavior of animals subjected to confinement (veal calves in stalls and laying hens in cages) were prompted by concerns for the humane treatment of animals and by the belief that stereotypies are indicators of mental suffering (Dantzer, 1986). These stereotypies are not arbitrary; they appear to develop from the early attempts of animals to escape from their enclosures. That is, behavioral patterns gradually become increasingly restricted and ultimately stereotypic.

Therefore, stereotypies may be serving either an arousal or de-arousal function for the organism. Studies performed using blood levels of cortisol or adrenocorticotropic hormones as an index of the general state of arousal have revealed that plasma levels of cortisol drop during performance of stereotypies (Brett & Levine, 1979; Dantzer & Mormede, 1983). Persons with Tourette's syndrome often report a buildup of stress when they suppress their tics that is dissipated when they permit them to reemerge (Lang, 1992).

Because both increases in arousal (such as anxiety or excitement) and decreases in arousal (such as sensory deprivation or boredom) may result in increased stereotypy, it is tempting to speculate that a homeostatic mechanism exists to maintain arousal level within a preferred range (Brett & Levine, 1979). It is conceivable that there is a survival value to the organism in the maintenance of an optimal level of arousal for effective response to changing environmental stressors.

Perhaps what is most clear from all of this information is that much ambiguity surrounds the definition of stereotypy. An abundance of terminology to describe movement (e.g., stereotypy, habit, mannerism, tic, dyskinesia) does not serve to clarify without precise criteria for differentiation. In a study that investigated the ability of blinded experienced raters to differentiate stereotypies from neuroleptic-related dyskinesias in children with autism, the movement disorders were not reliably differentiated from each other. The raters, psychiatrists with expertise in tardive dyskinesia or autism, tended to overdiagnose the finding with which they had more expertise (Meiselas, Spencer, Oberfield, Peselow, Angrist, & Campbell, 1989).

It is impossible to classify hyperkinetic movement disorders with regard to etiology by observation alone. For example, if you were observing a person who repeatedly bit his or her nails, you could make one of the following assessments: a normal developmental phase in a young child, a nervous habit in a teenager; a mannerism in a person with schizophrenia, or a stereotypy in a person with mental retardation or who is congenitally blind.

Therefore, a clinical categorization is largely based on the setting in which the repetitive movement is found. A motor behavior cannot be evaluated in isolation. The fundamentals of the person's history and clinical examination underlie an accurate diagnosis.

CONDITIONS ASSOCIATED WITH STEREOTYPY

Stereotyped behaviors are described in a number of heterogenous settings. Rhythmical stereotypes are observed in normally developing infants (Thelen, 1981). The appearance of these behaviors in different body locations (leg kicking, arm flapping) has been correlated with chronological age.

Over time, these coarse rhythmical movements evolve into coordinated, purposeful movement. They appear before the acquisition of specific developmental milestones, forming a bridge between uncoordinated motor activity and skillful voluntary motor control.

Stereotypies may reappear during early childhood in a variety of forms. Head banging, body rocking, hair twirling, or teeth grinding (bruxism) may occur transiently in children who are developing normally (Campbell, Grega, Green, & Bennett, 1983; Werry, Carlielle, & Fitzpatrick, 1983). These studies found that between 3% and 15% of children without disabilities engaged in head banging. Persistent body rocking was observed in approximately 20% of the children. These rhythmic movements have been variably interpreted as either discharging tension or providing a form of sensory comfort to the child. They are noted with increased frequency among children suffering from parental neglect; however, stereotypies are not uncommon among children without evidence of emotional disturbance. With advancing age and maturity, these developmental stereotypies gradually disappear, either spontaneously or due to conscious inhibition prompted by increasing social awareness.

Mental retardation, schizophrenia, and autism are frequently cited as conditions in which stereotypies are manifested. A 1987 study found that 34% of a sample of nonambulatory adults who were profoundly retarded exhibited at least one type of stereotypic behavior (Dura, Mulick, & Rasnake, 1987). An earlier study found the prevalence of stereotyped movements and postures to be two-thirds of the total population in a single residential institution serving persons with mental retardation (Berkson & Davenport, 1962). The presence of stereotypy was inversely correlated with IQ and directly correlated with length of institutionalization.

An association between the development of stereotyped behavior and the proximity to others manifesting stereotypy is implied by these data. Pigeons develop stereotypies at a higher rate when placed in visual contact with other birds displaying stereotyped behavior (Palya & Zacny, 1980). In addition, the incidence of tardive dyskinesia is higher in individuals who are institutionalized than in psychiatric outpatients, although this may simply reflect greater neuroleptic exposure (Weiner & Lang, 1989).

Stereotypies were well described in persons with schizophrenia prior to the introduction of neuroleptic agents, and they are most commonly associated with the catatonic form of schizophrenia. The abnormal movements range from simple motor behaviors to complex or bizarre gestures that are fraught with symbolism for the person. In one study, 24% of 250 persons with catatonic schizophrenia demonstrated stereotypic behavior (Morrison, 1973). A survey of 224 children with autism revealed that stereotypy was present in at least a mild form in the majority (Campbell et al., 1990). The presence of stereotypy was negatively correlated with IQ and positively correlated with overall symptomatology and severity of illness.

Stereotyped behaviors may be induced by a variety of pharmacologic agents that affect the dopaminergic pathways of the central nervous system (CNS). The long-term administration of levodopa or dopamine receptor agonists for Parkinson's disease commonly leads to the production of dyskinesias. Although these involuntary movements are often generalized and choreiform in nature, stereotypic oro-bucco-lingual dyskinesias are not uncommon. Reducing the dosage of dopaminergic agents reduces the dyskinesias; however, this results in an exacerbation of parkinsonian symptoms.

CNS stimulants such as amphetamines, pemoline, and methylphenidate may trigger repetitive motor behaviors by releasing dopamine from nerve terminals in the striatum. Cocaine may produce a similar effect by inhibiting synaptic uptake of dopamine, thereby increasing synaptic concentration.

The induction of stereotypy by amphetamines has been an area of intensive study. Both single high doses and repeated low doses of amphetamine will induce repetitive, persistent behaviors in a variety of animals. Interestingly, amphetamine-induced stereotyped behavior is species-specific or characteristic of the species of the animal (Klawans, Hitri, Nausieda, & Weiner, 1977; Weiner & Sanchez-Ramos, 1992). For example, a chewing, gnawing behavior has been observed in rats, whereas a repetitive pecking behavior has been seen in pigeons. These activities are characterized by a progressive narrowing of the animal's behavioral repertoire until a single behavior dominates.

Humans who abuse amphetamine intravenously exhibit a similar narrowing of behavior patterns. A wide variety of repetitive behaviors has been described, including compulsive shoe shining, perpetual bathing and grooming, or a preoccupation with cleaning and sorting belongings (Weiner & Sanchez-Ramos, 1992). Although a diversity of activities has been observed, the induced activity is specific and consistent for each amphetamine abuser. This behavior is called punding. Remarkably, these activities are described as pleasurable by the drug user, and attempts to interrupt these behaviors produce anxiety.

The concept of stereotypy as a dopamine-mediated behavior is the common thread that may account for the occurrence of these behaviors in a wide diversity of settings. The evidence that supports this concept is as follows. Pharmacologic agents with the ability to increase dopaminergic activity (e.g., amphetamine, methylphenidate, apomorphine, pemoline, cocaine, and levodopa) produce stereotyped behavior. Conversely, dopamine receptor antagonists (neuroleptics) or inhibition of dopamine synthesis with alpha-methyl-paratyrosine blocks the production of stereotypies by amphetamine.

Furthermore, the pharmacologic effects have been localized to the dopamine receptors of the corpus striatum. Stereotactic injection of dopamine into the neostriatum of rats produces stereotypies, whereas similar injection into extrastriatal CNS areas is ineffective. As might be anticipated, stereotactic injection of neuroleptic agents into the striatum prevents amphetamine-induced stereotyped behavior (Klawans & Weiner, 1974).

The induction of stereotypy is facilitated by the cumulative effect of the appropriate pharmacologic agent on an abnormal substrate. Extremely high doses of levodopa are required to produce stereotyped movements in normal monkeys, while more modest doses produce similar movements in monkeys with destructive lesions of both caudate nuclei. Similarly, chronic levodopa therapy is associated with the induction of dyskinesias in persons with Parkinson's disease, but not in healthy persons.

Although there is abundant evidence that stereotyped motor behaviors are regulated by the CNS dopamine pathways involved in the control of movement, other neurotransmitters modulate and influence the production of stereotypy, including cholinergic agents, serotonergic agents, and opiates. Cholinergic agents inhibit both amphetamine-induced stereotypy and hyperkinetic movement disorders, whereas anticholinergic agents have the opposite effects (Klawans & Weiner, 1974). Both serotonin agonists and antagonists have been demonstrated to suppress spontaneous stereotyped tongue protrusions in monkeys (Casey, 1992). Opiates also can induce stereotypies; however, naloxone, a specific blocker of opiate receptors, can both prevent and inhibit the dyskinetic syndromes associated with neuroleptic use (Pollock & Kornetsky, 1991).

Stereotyped behaviors are seen in a number of diverse settings in clinical neurology. Theoretically, any process that causes injury to the extrapyramidal system, in particular to the dopamine pathways of the basal ganglia and substantia nigra, has the potential to precipitate stereotypies. Traumatic injury, toxic–metabolic insults, genetic diseases, neurodegenerative disorders, vascular events, infectious processes, and neoplastic disease are all plausible etiologic conditions. In this chapter, three neurological disorders are presented in greater detail as examples of settings in which stereotypies are observed in clinical neurology: Rett's syndrome, Gilles de la Tourette's syndrome, and tardive dyskinesia.

Rett's Syndrome

Rett's syndrome was first described in children in 1966 by Andreas Rett. It is a progressive neurodegenerative disease reported to affect only females. The natural history of this disorder is particularly striking. Parents report normal physical and cognitive development in the first 6 to 18 months of life. However, this apparently normal period of development is followed by a period of stagnation and then a progressive loss of previously acquired cognitive and motor skills (Van Acker, 1991).

Regression occurs across all areas of development, including motor function, social interaction, and language skills. Interestingly, a characteristic finding in children with Rett's syndrome is the loss of purposeful use of the hands followed by the appearance of stereotypic hand movements (Nomura & Segawa, 1990). Between 1 and 3 years of age, a repetitive pattern of hand clasping, hand washing, and hand-to-mouth movements become a prominent symptom, and these movements are often virtually continuous during waking hours.

Developmental deterioration is also demonstrated by a deceleration of head growth and a stiff-legged, broad-based gait that sometimes results in the loss of ambulation. Intellectual function is severely compromised; these children are generally reported to fall within the severe-to-profound range of mental retardation. With advancing age, parkinsonian features such as bradykinesia, rigidity, and a loss of facial expressivity develop (Fitzgerald, Jankovic, & Percy, 1990).

Rett's syndrome is thought to be underrecognized; it is estimated that of a possible 10,000 cases in the United States, only about 10% have been identified thus far. A lack of awareness of this disorder and a tendency to confuse it with infantile autism contribute to its underreporting. The development of profound mental retardation, the progressive difficulties with ambulation, and the stereotypic hand movements are some of the characteristics of Rett's that distinguish it from autism.

The etiology is not known; however, Rett's syndrome appears to be a genetic disorder, as demonstrated in twin studies. The pathogenesis remains unclear, but the leading hypothesis is that the motor dysfunction results from alterations of the dopamine pathways of the extrapyramidal system. Unfortunately, therapeutic trials with a variety of dopaminergic agents have been disappointing, with no consistent effects demonstrated on either the symptomatology or the disease progress.

Gilles de la Tourette's Syndrome

Tourette's syndrome was described by George Gilles de la Tourette in 1885. His description included most of the characteristic features—the waxing and waning of multiple motor and vocal tics, the early age of onset, the importance of hereditary factors, and the chronic nature of the disorder (Goetz & Klawans, 1982). Although more than a century has passed, Tourette's syndrome continues to be misunderstood and underrecognized.

Studies of persons with Tourette's have revealed that the most common motor tics are eye blinking, facial grimacing, and head jerking; the most prevalent vocal tics are throat clearing, grunting, and sniffing (Comings & Comings, 1985; Jankovic & Rohaidy, 1987). Some form of phonic or vocal tic is required for a diagnosis of Tourette's syndrome. Coprolalia (involuntary usage of obscene language) is often mistakenly considered a common manifestation of Tourette's. A recent survey of 112 younger individuals with Tourette's revealed that only 8% of the group exhibited coprolalia (Goldenberg, Brown, & Weiner, 1994).

There is evidence to suggest that Tourette's syndrome is related to altered CNS dopaminergic function. Dopaminergic agents may precipitate or exacerbate Tourette's symptoms, whereas blockade of dopamine pathways decreases the frequency and severity of tics.

A provocative hypothesis for the pathogenesis of Tourette's syndrome proposes that the brain regions involved in Tourette's, specifically the basal ganglia and limbic system, are the phylogenetic counterparts in humans of the regions that functioned in primitive reproductive behavior (Kurlan, 1992a). From an evolutionary standpoint, these areas would have been responsible for vestigial reproductive motor programs such as mating dances and sexual foreplay, as well as vestigial vocal programs such as mating songs and noises. A disinhibition of these primitive neural systems might underlie the peculiar motor and vocal tics observed in Tourette's syndrome.

Treatment is often not warranted for the large number of persons who are mildly affected by Tourette's syndrome. Education and supportive counseling for the individual, his or her family members, and school personnel often eliminate the need for medication. Medications such as clonazepam, clonidine, and neuroleptics may be helpful for those individuals whose symptoms are moderate or severe. Although neuroleptics are generally the most efficacious, they are also associated with significant adverse effects. Therefore, trials of clonazepam or clonidine should be attempted first. When neuroleptics such as haloperidol are required, 66% to 80% of individuals with Tourette's demonstrate improvement (Jankovic & Rohaidy, 1987; Shapiro, Shapiro, & Sweet, 1981). However, chronic neuroleptic therapy carries the risk of inducing tardive dyskinesia, a condition that may be difficult to recognize in its early stages in individuals with Tourette's who have facial tics.

Tardive Dyskinesia

The delayed onset of an involuntary movement disorder following neuroleptic exposure was first recognized and described in the late 1950s, several years after the introduction of chlorpromazine, the first neuroleptic agent. The prerequisites for a diagnosis of tardive dyskinesia (TD) are a history of at least 3 months of neuroleptic exposure, the presence of involuntary movements, and the absence of other conditions that might produce a movement disorder. However, the simplicity of these criteria belies the difficulties that may be encountered when considering this diagnosis.

Abnormal movements with similarity to tardive dyskinesia were described in persons with schizophrenia before the introduction of neuroleptics, although the mannerisms associated with schizophrenia are less rhythmic in nature, more complex, and highly ritualistic (Cunningham, Owens, Johnstone, & Frith, 1982; Morrison, 1973; Rogers & Hymas, 1988). Furthermore, dyskinetic movements, particularly in the orofacial region, may occur spontaneously in older persons (Weiner & Klawans, 1973). The prevalence of spontaneous lingual–facial–buccal dyskinesias in older persons has been found to be between 8% and 10%.

Neuroleptic medications may also induce acute dystonic reactions or acute transient dyskinesias, particularly when treatment is initiated or when the dosage is changed. These events are distinct from a diagnosis of tardive dyskinesia, although they may identify a subgroup of persons who are more at risk for future extrapyramidal syndromes (Keepers & Casey, 1991).

A variety of abnormal involuntary movements have been described with tardive dyskinesia: chorea (irregular, brief movements that flow from one body part to another), athetosis (slower, sinuous, writhing movements), dystonias (slower, more sustained postures), and akathesia (a subjective sensation of restlessness associated with an inability to sit still). In spite of the range of these movements, tardive dyskinesia is often cited as a prototype of stereotypic behavior.

In fact, some researchers consider the chorea associated with tardive dyskinesia to be less random and unpredictable, and more stereotypic and repetitive, than the movements of other choreiform disorders, such as

Huntington's disease (Kurlan, 1992b). Stereotyped movements are particularly characteristic of oro-bucco-lingual dyskinesias—often the earliest and sometimes the sole feature of TD. Fine, vermicular movements of the tongue progress to to-and-fro lateral movements and then to twisting or curling tongue movements with bulging of the cheek and involuntary tongue protrusions. Limb dyskinesias also are often stereotypic with twisting, piano-playing–like movements of fingers and toes, foot tapping, and marching in place.

It is difficult to characterize the natural history of TD. The onset is usually insidious, and the symptoms are often complicated by adjustments and variations in medication regimens from person to person. Long-term data indicate that after a period of progression, the movements begin to stabilize or gradually improve, even in those persons who continue on neuroleptics (Casey, Povisen, Meidahl, & Gerlach, 1986). It may take 3 to 5 years for the symptoms to abate after the withdrawal of neuroleptic treatment. In a minority of instances, the dyskinesias persist. It is unclear at this time whether this is actually permanent TD or persistent dyskinesias in that group of individuals who are predisposed to develop spontaneous dyskinesias (Marsden, 1985).

The CNS dopamine pathways have been implicated in the production of the stereotyped movements of TD. Yet even though neuroleptic agents ameliorate the stereotypy of Tourette's syndrome, they are the etiologic factor in tardive dyskinesia. The most widely accepted hypothesis is that chronic dopaminergic blockade due to long-term neuroleptic administration results in a drug-induced denervation of the postsynaptic dopamine receptor. Eventually, a condition of postsynaptic receptor supersensitivity evolves and the movement disorder appears. Consequently, TD is often first noted when the neuroleptic dosage is reduced or discontinued.

Because the treatment of tardive dyskinesia is difficult and often inadequate, the major emphasis is on prevention. The indications for long-term antipsychotic treatment must be clearly established and regularly reevaluated. Neuroleptics should be administered in the lowest possible dosage, with low potency preparations used when feasible. Treatment

29

should include routine examination for the early signs of TD, particularly the fine, vermicular movements of the tongue. Reversal of TD is most likely to occur when neuroleptics are discontinued at the earliest sign of the appearance of the movement disorder. Whether TD is related to duration of neuroleptic treatment or total dosage of neuroleptic administered has not yet been determined.

Once TD is diagnosed, neuroleptics should be gradually withdrawn if the psychiatric condition permits. The severity of the movement disorder may also limit the speed with which neuroleptic dosages can be tapered. Clonazepam and other benzodiazepines may reduce the severity of dyskinesias, but the most effective agents for symptomatic relief are dopamine antagonists. Naturally, it is difficult to rationalize the use of increasing dosages of the etiologic agent to control the symptoms. Therefore, presynaptic dopamine depleting agents, such as reserpine, are often used with some success.

TOWARD AN UNDERSTANDING OF STEREOTYPY

The wide range of heterogenous conditions that give rise to stereotyped behavior is in contrast to the more narrow and redundant repertoire of stereotypies that are produced in such diverse settings. Whether it is the animal model of amphetamine-induced stereotypy, the mannerisms associated with schizophrenia, the purposeless repetitive behaviors associated with mental retardation, the tics associated with Tourette's syndrome, or the persistent dyskinesias following neuroleptic use, similar and analogous motor behaviors with a special affinity for the face and mouth have been observed.

The common denominator may be the presence of preprogrammed neuronal circuits in the brainstem and possibly the basal ganglia that give rise to primitive and stereotyped motor functions in man (Guyton, 1987). Newborns without higher brain structures (anencephalia) are able to perform numerous motor functions such as sucking, sticking out their tongue, moving their hands to their mouth to suck their fingers, and crying, most likely because of the presence of hard-wired intrinsic motor patterning.

Therefore, stereotypies may be primitive, phylogenetically older motor programs that are unmasked when higher cortical functions are interrupted. They are appropriately demonstrated during infancy before the development of complex cortical pathways, and they have been noted to persist in ill babies who are ultimately developmentally retarded.

The dopamine pathways of the extrapyramidal system play a regulatory role in the production of organized patterned movement, and derangement of these pathways may trigger the overexpression of programmed motor behaviors. Although it has been previously postulated that stereotyped behavior plays an adaptive role as a regulator of arousal homeostasis, it cannot be ruled out that stereotypies are simply the spontaneous behavioral output of disregulated neural pathways and disinhibited primitive motor programs (Dantzer, 1986; Lewis, Baumeister, & Mailman, 1987; Thelen, 1981).

This chapter has explored the defining features of stereotypies, the clinical conditions in which they are observed, and the theoretical constructs that may explain their expression. Presently, the classification of stereotyped behavior continues to be based on description and is not yet rooted in clear anatomic or pathophysiologic principles. Given the variability of human pathology, the concept of stereotypy should continue to be broadly defined to be most clinically useful.

REFERENCES

Berkson, G., & Davenport, R. K. (1962). Stereotyped movements of mental defectives: I. Initial survey. *American Journal of Mental Deficiency, 66,* 849–852.

Berkson, G., & Gallagher, R. J. (1986). Control of feedback from abnormal stereotyped behaviors. In M. G. Wade (Ed.), *The development of coordination, control and skill in the mentally handicapped* (pp. 7–24). Amsterdam: North Holland.

Brett, L. P., & Levine, S. (1979). Schedule induced polydipsia suppresses pituitary-adrenal activity in rats. *Journal of Comparative and Physiological Psychology, 93,* 946–956.

Campbell, M., Grega, D. M., Green, W. H., & Bennett, W. G. (1983). Neuroleptic-induced dyskinesias in children. *Clinical Neuropharmacology, 6,* 207–222.

Campbell, M., Locascio, J. J., Choroco, M. C., Spencer, E. K., Malone, R. P., Kafanteris, V., & Overall, J. E. (1990). Stereotypies and tardive dyskinesia: Abnormal movements in autistic children. *Psychopharmacology Bulletin, 26,* 260–266.

Casey, D. E. (1992, October 3). *Neuroleptic drug-induced extrapyramidal syndromes in non-human primates: Implications for understanding brain-behavior relationships.* Paper presented at the Conference on Stereotypies: Brain–behavior relationships, University of Illinois, Urbana, IL.

Casey, D. E., Povisen, V. J., Meidahl, B., & Gerlach, J. (1986). Neuroleptic induced tardive dyskinesia and parkinsonism: Changes during several years of continuing treatment. *Psychopharmacology Bulletin, 22,* 250–253.

Comings, D. E., & Comings, B. G. (1985). Tourette's syndrome: Clinical and psychological aspects of 250 cases. *American Journal of Human Genetics, 37,* 435–450.

Cunningham, J., Owens, D. G., Johnstone, E. C., & Frith, C. D. (1982). Spontaneous involuntary disorders of movement. *Archives of General Psychiatry, 39,* 452–461.

Dantzer, R. (1986). Behavioral, physiological and functional aspects of stereotyped behavior: A review and a reinterpretation. *Journal of Animal Science, 62,* 1776–1786.

Dantzer, R., & Mormede, P. (1983). Dearousal properties of stereotyped behavior: Evidence from pituitary–adrenal correlates in pigs. *Applied Animal Ethology, 10,* 233.

Dura, J. R., Mulick, J. A., & Rasnake, L. K. (1987). Prevalence of stereotypy among institutionalized nonambulatory profoundly mentally retarded people. *American Journal of Mental Deficiency, 91,* 548–549.

Fitzgerald, P. M., Jankovic, J., & Percy, A. K. (1990). Rett syndrome and associated movement disorders. *Movement Disorders, 5,* 195–202.

Goetz, C. G., & Klawans, H. L. (1982). Gilles de la Tourette on Tourette syndrome. In A. J. Friedhoff & T. N. Chase (Eds.), *Gilles de la Tourette Syndrome* (pp. 1–16). New York: Raven Press.

Goldenberg, J. N., Brown, S. B., & Weiner, W. J. (1994). Coprolalia in younger patients with Gilles de la Tourette syndrome. *Movement Disorders, 9,* 622–625.

Guyton, A. C. (1987). Motor functions of the brainstem and basal ganglia. *Basic neuroscience.* Philadelphia: W. B. Saunders.

Jankovic, J., & Rohaidy, H. (1987). Motor, behavioral and pharmacologic findings in Tourette's syndrome. *The Canadian Journal of Neurological Sciences, 14,* 541–546.

Keepers, G. A., & Casey, D. E. (1991). Use of neuroleptic-induced extrapyramidal symptoms to predict future vulnerability to side effects. *American Journal of Psychiatry, 148,* 85–89.

Klawans, H. L., Hitri, A., Nausieda, P. A., & Weiner, W. J. (1977). Animal models of dyskinesia. In I. Hanin & E. Usdin (Eds.), *Animal models in psychiatry and neurology* (pp. 351–364). New York and Oxford: Pergamon Press.

Klawans, H. L., & Weiner, W. J. (1974). Animal models of human extrapyramidal disorders. In H. L. Klawans (Ed.), *Models of human neurological diseases* (pp. 5–38). Amsterdam: Excerpta Medica.

Koegel, R. L., & Covert, A. (1972). The relationship of self-stimulation to learning in autistic children. *Journal of Applied Behavior Analysis, 5,* 381–387.

Kurlan, R. (1992a). The pathogenesis of Tourette's syndrome. *Archives of Neurology, 49,* 874–876.

Kurlan, R. (1992b). Spontaneous movement disorders in psychiatric patients. In A. E. Lang & W. J. Weiner (Eds.), *Drug-induced movement disorders* (pp. 257–280). Mt. Kisco, NY: Futura.

Lang, A. E. (1992). Clinical phenomenology of tic disorders: Selected aspects. In T. N. Chase, A. J. Friedhoff, & D. J. Cohen (Eds.), *Advances in neurology, 58,* (pp. 25–32). New York: Raven Press.

Lewis, M. H., Baumeister, A. A., & Mailman, R. B. (1987). A neurobiological alternative to the perceptual reinforcement hypothesis of stereotyped behavior: A commentary on "self-stimulatory behavior and perceptual reinforcement." *Journal of Applied Behavior Analysis, 20,* 253–258.

Marsden, C. D. (1985). Is tardive dyskinesia a unique disorder? In D. E. Casey, T. N. Chase, E. Christensen, & J. Gerlach (Eds.), *Dyskinesia—Research and treatment* (pp. 64–71). *Psychopharmacology* (Suppl. 2). Berlin Heidelberg: Springer-Verlag.

Meiselas, K. D., Spencer, E. K., Oberfield, R., Peselow, E. D., Angrist, B., & Campbell, M. (1989). Differentiation of stereotypies from neuroleptic-related dyskinesias in autistic children. *Journal of Clinical Psychopharmacology, 9,* 207–209.

Morrison, J. R. (1973). Catatonia. *Archives of General Psychiatry, 28,* 39–41.

Newell, K. M., Van Emmerik, R. E. A., & Sprague, R. L. (1992). Stereotypy and variability. In M. Newell & D. M. Corcus (Eds.), *Variability and motor control* (pp. 475–496). Champaign, IL: Human Kinetics.

Nomura, Y., & Segawa, M. (1990). Characteristics of motor disturbances of the Rett syndrome. *Brain and Development, 12,* 27–30.

Palya, W. L., & Zacny, J. P. (1980). Stereotyped adjunctive pecking by caged pigeons. *Animal Learned Behavior, 8,* 293.

Pollock, J., & Kornetsky, C. (1991). Naloxone prevents and blocks the emergence of neuroleptic-mediated oral stereotypic behaviors. *Neuropsychopharmacology, 4,* 245–249.

Rogers, D., & Hymas, N. (1988). Sporadic facial stereotypies in patients with schizophrenia and compulsive disorders. In J. Jankovic & E. Tolosa (Eds.), *Advances in neurology* (Vol. 49, pp. 383–394). New York: Raven Press.

Shapiro, A. K., Shapiro, E., & Sweet, R. D. (1981). Treatment of tics and Tourette's syndrome. In A. Barbeau (Ed.), *Disorders of movement* (pp. 105–132). Lancaster, England: MTP Press.

Silverstein, S. M., Como, P. G., Palumbo, D., West, L., & Kurlan, R. (1992, October 18–22). *A comparison of impaired attention in adult Tourette's syndrome and Attention Deficit Disorder patients.* Poster session at the Annual Meeting of the American Neurological Association, Toronto, Ontario, Canada.

Thelen, E. (1981). Rhythmical behavior in infancy: An ethological perspective. *Developmental Psychology, 17,* 237–257.

Van Acker, R. (1991). Rett syndrome: A review of current knowledge. *Journal of Autism and Developmental Disorders, 21,* 381–406.

Weiner, W. J., & Klawans, H. L. (1973). Lingual–facial–buccal movements in the elderly. I: Pathophysiology and treatment. II: Pathogenesis and relationship to senile chorea. *Journal of the American Geriatrics Society, 21,* 314–320.

Weiner, W. J., & Lang, A. E. (1989). *Movement disorders: A comprehensive survey.* Mt. Kisco, NY: Futura.

Weiner, W. J., & Sanchez-Ramos, J. R. (1992). Movement disorders and dopaminomimetic stimulant drugs. In A. E. Lang & W. J. Weiner (Eds.), *Drug-induced movement disorders* (pp. 315–337). Mt. Kisco, NY: Futura.

Werry, J. A., Carlielle, J., & Fitzpatrick, J. (1983). Rhythmic motor activities (stereotypies) in children under five: Etiology and prevalence. *Journal of American Academy of Child Psychiatry, 22,* 329–336.

PART TWO

Understanding the Causes

3

Neurobiological Basis of Stereotyped Movement Disorder

Mark H. Lewis, John P. Gluck, James W. Bodfish,
Alan J. Beauchamp, and Richard B. Mailman

Stereotyped behavior involves rhythmic and topographically invariant motor acts that occur without obvious eliciting stimuli and have no clearly established function for the biological organism (Lewis & Baumeister, 1982; Ridley & Baker, 1982). The rhythmic and topographically invariant nature of stereotypies has been strikingly depicted in analog tracings of the stereotyped body rocking displayed by individuals with mental retardation, transduced using a single plane accelerometer (see Lewis et al., 1984). Berkson (1983) has argued that the rhythmic or periodic nature of stereotyped behavior may be its most dramatic feature. The apparent "purposelessness" or lack of function of stereotyped behavior, although at the heart of its definition, is less easy to establish, however. Many functions have been posited for stereotypies, including reward, stress reduction, sensory stimulation, and amelioration of an impoverished environment (see recent reviews by Mason, 1991). Some evidence exists to support all of these hypothesized functions. For example, the persistence of stereotypies, even in the face of aversive consequences, has been taken by some as evidence of the rewarding nature of the behavior. Indeed, there

Preparation of this chapter was supported, in part, by Public Health Service Grant HD 30615.

is some evidence that the sensory stimulation provided by stereotyped movements may be reinforcing in humans (Lovaas, Newsom, & Hickman, 1987). Stereotypies have been posited to increase arousal (Hutt, Hutt, Lee, & Ousted, 1964) or reduce stress (Brett & Levine, 1979). The observation that the removal of the opportunity to engage in a stereotyped behavior in animals (e.g., scheduled induced water licking) is associated with increased pituitary–adrenal axis activity has been confirmed by several groups (see Mason, 1991). The functional consequences of stereotypy for the organism are far from firmly established, however, and conclusions drawn by various theorists rely on correlative data or assumptions that have not been rigorously tested (see, for example, Lewis, Baumeister, & Mailman, 1987). Moreover, stereotypy is a descriptive term, not a behavior. As such, stereotyped behavior can, and probably is, maintained by multiple functions. Different environmental functions do not necessitate different biologies, however, and stereotypies may be related to a common pathophysiology.

Stereotyped behavior can be observed in many species in a variety of experimental and natural contexts (Lewis & Baumeister, 1982). Ethologists, in analyzing displacement activities in animals and humans, have described highly stereotyped sequences of behavior in response to such motivational conditions as frustration and conflict (e.g., Duncan & Wood-Gush, 1972). Stereotypies appear in the repertoire of all normally developing children, exhibiting a clear developmental sequence (Thelen, 1981). More frequently, however, stereotyped behavior is thought to represent a decreased ability to respond adaptively to a changing environment (Isaacson & Gispen, 1990), and thus is considered to be abnormal and often taken as evidence of a dysregulated central nervous system (CNS). This is because stereotyped behavior is a frequent consequence of abnormal rearing conditions (Berkson, 1967), impoverished environments (Levy, 1944; Meyer-Holzapfel, 1968), frustration or conflict (Fentress, 1976), administration of high or chronic doses of certain psychotropic drugs (Ellinwood, 1967), or brain injury, particularly in development (Baumeister & Forehand, 1973). Thus, stereotypies represent an important model for studying brain–behavior relationships, particularly following CNS insult (Cooper & Dourish, 1990). One important avenue for understanding the nature of stereotyped behavior, its role in functional adaptation, and (in the case of certain clinical populations) its treatment is the conduct of basic studies aimed at elucidating the neurobiological mechanisms that mediate its expression.

This chapter reviews our findings relevant to the neurobiology of stereotyped behavior and the implications of these and related observations to treatment of stereotyped movement disorder in humans. Some of the information relevant to this topic comes from psychopharmacological studies in rodents, in which drugs were used that alter central dopamine transmission. Thus, our work in this area is reviewed, as are other relevant studies that implicate specific neurotransmitters in the mediation of stereotypies. We also discuss our progress in studying the neurobiological basis of stereotyped behavior observed in rhesus monkeys that underwent early social deprivation. For reasons to be presented, we believe that this is a very useful animal model for studying the neurobiological basis of stereotyped behavior in persons with severe mental retardation and autism. Stereotyped and self-injurious behavior are invariant consequences of such early differential social experience in rhesus monkeys (Goosen, 1981). Furthermore, as will be discussed, the stereotyped behavior seen in early socially deprived monkeys meets multiple important criteria necessary for a useful animal model of the pathological stereotypies observed in humans. Finally, we describe some preliminary studies designed to test the hypothesis of altered central dopamine and serotonin systems in those individuals with mental retardation who engage in high rates of stereotyped behavior. These experiments are reviewed in terms of their relationship to studies of the efficacy of various pharmacologic treatments of stereotyped behavior in this population.

THE NEUROPHARMACOLOGY OF STEREOTYPED BEHAVIOR

Dopamine Agonist–Induced Stereotypy

Starting in the early 1960s, highly stereotyped sequences of behavior were reported in individuals abusing psychostimulants such as amphetamine.

These behaviors included repetion of the same phrase over and over again, repeated assembling and disassembling of objects, repetitive sorting of the contents of a handbag, or repetitive mouth and tongue movements (Ellinwood, 1967, 1969; Rylander, 1971). The induction of stereotyped behaviors in individuals who abuse stimulants was part of a syndrome that resembled paranoid psychosis. Because the actions of stimulants could mimic some of the features of schizophrenia, considerable attention was given to the effects of these compounds in experimental animals. It is now well established that stereotyped patterns of behavior can be induced in a number of mammalian species following stimulant administration (Randrup & Munkvad, 1967). In addition, stereotypies can be induced in rodents or nonhuman primates through the administration of drugs like apomorphine that act directly on dopamine receptors and by the dopamine precursor L-dopa (Fog, 1972; Lewis, Baumeister, McCorkle, & Mailman, 1985).

Related experiments have established the importance of the nigrostriatal dopamine pathway by showing that dopamine or a dopamine agonist injected into the corpus striatum induced stereotyped behavior in rats (e.g., Ernst & Smelik, 1966). The corpus striatum is the terminal field for the major dopamine pathway that has its cell bodies in substantia nigra and sends ascending projections to striatum. Induction of stereotyped behavior by application of gamma-aminobutyric acid (GABA) agonists to the substantia nigra pars reticulata supports the importance of the nigrostriatal circuitry and its output pathways, including the reciprocal GABA-mediated descending strionigral pathway (Scheel-Kruger, Arnt, Braestrup, Christensen, Cools, & Maglund, 1978; Scheel-Kruger, Arnt, Magelund, Olianas, Przewlocka, & Christensen, 1980). Similarly, lesions of the superior colliculus, an important target of descending nigral projections, decrease the ability of dopamine agonists to induce stereotypy, a finding that provides additional support for the importance of this neural circuit (Redgrave, Dean, Donohue, & Pope, 1980). Not surprisingly, dopamine agonist–induced stereotyped behavior can be blocked by dopamine receptor antagonists such as haloperidol (Ridley, Baker, & Scraggs, 1979). Indeed, blockade of amphetamine- or apomorphine-induced stereotyped behavior became an important screen for compounds with potential antipsychotic activity (Janssen, Niemegeers, & Schellekens, 1965; Janssen, Niemegeers, Schellekens, & Leanerts, 1967).

Amphetamine-induced stereotypy is believed to be dependent upon the ability of this psychostimulant to release dopamine in the nervous system. Consistent with this idea, these stereotypies can be blocked by inhibiting the synthesis of dopamine (e.g., by pretreating with alpha-methyl-p-tyrosine) or destroying presynaptic dopamine terminals (e.g., using the neurotoxicant 6-hydroxydopamine). Conversely, cytochemical lesioning of dopamine pathways using 6-hydroxydopamine makes animals more sensitive (i.e., showing effects at lower doses) to direct-acting dopamine agonists such as apomorphine. This behavioral supersensitivity is particularly apparent in rats treated neonatally with 6-hydroxydopamine, as they exhibit intense stereotyped and self-injurious behavior when treated with apomorphine (Creese & Iversen, 1973; Ungerstedt, 1971). In our studies, rats having bilateral lesions of the substantia nigra induced by 6-OHDA (hydroxydopamine) responded to a low dose of apomorphine (0.3 mg/kg) with either a high degree of stereotyped grooming or gnawing and nose poking at the cage floor. In one case, the stereotyped grooming progressed to bouts of self-injurious behavior. Sham-lesioned rats treated with the same dose showed only sniffing and intermittent licking of the cage floor (Mileson, Lewis, & Mailman, 1991).

Dopamine Receptor Multiplicity and Stereotyped Behavior

If induction of stereotyped behavior is linked to stimulation or alterations of dopamine receptors, then the question of which receptor subtype(s) mediates this response becomes important. Recent efforts by molecular neurobiologists have resulted in the cloning of at least five different dopamine receptor subtypes. Based on pharmacologic, functional, and molecular biological similarities, these subtypes can be organized into two classes: "D_1-like" or "D_2-like," following nomenclature first proposed more than a decade ago (Garau, Govoni, Stefanini, Trabucchi, & Spano, 1978; Kebabian & Calne, 1979). D_1-like receptors are thought to mediate dopamine-induced increases in adenylate cyclase activity, whereas D_2-like receptor activation typically inhibits the activity of this enzyme (for reviews, see Andersen et al., 1990; Clark & White, 1987). Thus, the recently cloned dopamine receptor subtypes D_3 and D_4 are considered D_2-like, whereas the D_5 receptor is classified as D_1-like. Historically, the D_2 receptor was believed to be the site of action of most psychopharmacologic effects of numerous classes of both dopamine agonists and antagonists, including induction and blockade of stereotyped behavior (Creese, Sibley, Hamblin, & Leff, 1983). In 1984, however, we reported that the D_1 antagonist SCH23390 could potently inhibit apomorphine-induced stereotyped behavior and amphetamine-induced locomotion in rats, behaviors heretofore believed to be largely or exclusively D_2 receptor–mediated (Mailman, Schulz, Lewis, Staples, Rollema & Dehaven, 1984). This initial report of the ability of D_1 receptors to affect D_2 receptor function was soon confirmed (Molloy & Waddington, 1984), and the importance of D_1/D_2 receptor interactions in the production of stereotypies and other behavior is now widely appreciated (Arnt, Huttel, & Perregard, 1987; Bordi & Meller, 1989; Braun & Chase, 1986; Mashurano & Waddington, 1986; Meller, Bordi, & Bohmaker, 1988).

Despite this, the relative importance of D_1-like versus D_2-like receptors in the induction of stereotypies has been difficult to evaluate because, until recently, all available D_1 agonists (e.g., SKF38393) have had only partial functional efficacy. (In brain tissue, SKF38393 can cause only about half the maximal effect of dopamine in stimulating cAMP synthesis, a marker for this receptor.) Thus, the failure of SKF38393 to induce stereotyped behavior in rodents may indicate a lesser role for this receptor subtype or, perhaps more parsimoniously, the lack of a pharmacologic probe with the requisite efficacy. To complicate the issue further, most of the available mixed-direct agonists (like apomorphine or bromocriptine) appear to have both agonist and antagonist properties at D_1 receptors.

It has been reported that the synthesis and characterization of dihydrexidine, a hexahydrobenzo[a]phenanthridine was not only several-fold more potent in radioreceptor assays than SKF38393, but also was equally efficacious as dopamine in stimulating cAMP synthesis in striatal membranes (Brewster et al., 1990; Lovenberg et al., 1989). This made dihydrexidine the first bioavailable, full-efficacy D_1 agonist, and, as such, a powerful psychopharmacologic tool (Mottola, Brewster, Cook, Nichols, & Mailman, 1992). Interestingly, despite its significant D_1 potency, dihydrexidine also has some D_2 potency, being about tenfold selective for D_1 (i.e., [^{3}H]-SCH23390) vs. D_2 (i.e., [^{3}H]-spiperone) binding sites. Darney, Lewis, Brewster, Nichols, and Mailman (1991) tested the dose-dependent effects of dihydrexidine on the unconditioned motor behavior of rats. The results of this study indicated that, although dihydrexidine dose-dependently stimulated grooming, locomotion, and sniffing, there was little evidence of the highly stereotyped sequences of behavior typically observed following administration of mixed agonists. Thus, while the D_1 antagonist SCH23390 can potently block drug-induced stereotyped behavior, a selective, full-efficacy agonist shows little ability to induce such behavior.

Selective and potent D_2 antagonists have been reported to be efficacious in the inhibition of apomorphine-induced stereotypy. Moreover, the induction of highly stereotyped sequences of behavior has been reported following selective D_2 agonists (Waddington, Malloy, O'Boyle, & Pugh, 1990). Thus, there is strong evidence that D_2 receptors play a critical role in the induction and antagonism of stereotyped behavior. Assessment of the role played by other dopamine receptor subtypes must await the development of ligands selective for those sites.

Neurotransmitter Interactions in the Mediation of Stereotyped Behavior

Indirect- and direct-acting dopamine agonists have been the major focus of studies designed to elucidate the neurobiology of stereotyped behavior; however, complex behaviors typically involve polysynaptic circuitry that makes use of multiple transmitter systems. Thus, pharmacologic agents that interact with nondopaminergic receptors have also been shown to induce stereotypies (Lewis & Baumeister, 1982). These include compounds that interact with opioid, serotonin (5-HT), GABA, acetylcholine, and adenosine receptors.

Direct injections of either morphine or β-endorphin into the substantia nigra have resulted in intense stereotypies in rats. Similarly, chronic administration of the opiate agonists morphine or methadone results in both stereotyped and self-mutilative behavior in rodents (Iwamoto & Way, 1977). Opiate antagonists have also been reported to inhibit certain forms of stereotypy in movement-restricted farm animals (Dantzer, 1986). While opiate antagonists have been reported to be efficacious in treating self-injurious behavior in some cases, insufficient evidence exists to draw conclusions regarding their effectiveness in treating stereotypies in individuals with either mental retardation or autism (Sandman, Baron, & Weman, 1990). A substantial amount of literature exists detailing the close interaction between opioid and dopamine systems. Dense concentrations of opioid peptides and their receptors are found in terminal fields receiving innervation by dopamine neurons (e.g., striatum). There are also important enkephalin projections to substantia nigra and ventral tegmental area, nuclei of origin of the major dopamine pathways in the brain. Thus, opiate–dopamine interactions appear to mediate many of the effects already described.

Administration of the 5-HT precursor, 5-hydroxytryptophan, as well as drugs that either inhibit the uptake or facilitate the release of 5-HT, or act as direct 5-HT agonists, have been reported to induce a complex behavioral syndrome that includes stereotyped head weaving and forepaw treading (Curzon, 1990). Several lines of evidence suggest that these behaviors are dependent on 5-HT_{1A} receptors and the interactions of these receptors with dopamine systems. For example, head weaving and forepaw treading are blocked both by lesions of the nigrostriatal and mesolimbic dopamine pathways and by administration of the dopamine blocker, haloperidol.

Stereotyped behavior associated with administration of anticholinergic drugs has been reported in both humans and laboratory animals (Kulik & Wilbur, 1982). No doubt these observations involve modulation of a polysynaptic circuit that involves dopamine projections from substantia nigra (pars compacta) to striatal cholinergic interneurons expressing D_2 receptors. These interneurons, in turn, synapse on GABA cells that project either back to substantia nigra or to globus pallidus. Modulation of striatal dopamine function by anticholinergics is thought to be the basis for their efficacy in treating drug-induced parkinsonsim.

Stereotyped behavior has also been induced by activation of striatal efferent pathways, including projections to substantia nigra (pars reticulata) and globus pallidus. The importance of these GABAergic outflow pathways has been established by Scheel-Kruger et al. (1978, 1980). They demonstrated induction of stereotypies following administration of GABA agonists into either the striatum or substantia nigra. More distally, nigro-tectal pathways appear to mediate aspects of dopamine agonist–induced stereotypy. For example, lesions of the superior colliculus abolish apomorphine and amphetamine-induced stereotypy (Pope, Dean, & Redgrave, 1980; Redgrave et al., 1980).

Finally, methylxanthines, such as caffeine or theophylline also have been shown to induce stereotyped, and in high doses, self-injurious behavior in rodents. The mechanism of action of these pharmacodynamic effects appears to be blockade of adenosine receptors that are found in high concentrations in striatum. Recent evidence points to a strong interaction between A_2 adenosine receptors and D_2 dopamine receptors. The interaction between these striatal receptor subtypes is thought to be the mechanism mediating the psychomotor stimulant effects of methylxanthines (Ferre, Von Euler, Johansson, Fredholm, & Fuxe, 1991).

STEREOTYPED BEHAVIOR INDUCED BY EARLY SOCIAL DEPRIVATION OF RHESUS MONKEYS

Social deprivation during early development has profound effects on behavior of certain species of nonhuman primates (Harlow, Dodsworth, & Harlow, 1965). A defining feature of what has been termed the isolate syndrome is stereotyped behavior. The stereotyped behavior seen in rhesus monkeys following early social deprivation shares important properties with stereotypies observed in clinical populations. The topographies or forms of the behavior are strikingly similar. In each case, the behavioral abnormality is due to a developmental insult, persists through the lifetime of the organism, and is spontaneous in the repertoire of the individual (i.e., does not require a pharmacologic or environmental challenge). Finally, as we will establish later in this chapter, each appears to have similar neurobiological mechanisms.

We have been studying a group of rhesus monkeys that were reared without access to mother or peers during the first 6 or 9 months of their first year of life. Because this particular group of animals was almost 20 years of age at the initiation of this project, we were provided with the rare opportunity to study the long-term effects of early social deprivation on brain and behavior. One important focus of our studies has been to understand what neurobiological changes might be mediating the stereotyped behavior observed in these animals. Our working hypothesis has been that early social deprivation resulted in a loss of dopamine innervation to striatal areas with a consequent dopamine receptor supersensitivity.

Sensory Gating

Although the deleterious effects of early social deprivation on social and affective functioning in rhesus monkeys were clear, the effect of differential rearing on cognitive function had not been established. This question remained largely unanswered because of the difficulty in ascribing performance deficits on various tasks to cognitive function versus a host of other factors, such as arousal, hyperreactivity, movement disorders, and other potential artifacts. We (Beauchamp, Gluck, & Lewis, 1991) tested the effects of early social deprivation using a simple associative learning task. The use of this paradigm permitted the assessment of associative learning in socially deprived versus socially reared monkeys while only requiring the simplest response from the animal. This paradigm also allowed us to test for sensory-gating deficits that have been shown to result from alterations in central dopamine function.

The associative conditioning paradigm used has been referred to both as blocking and as the Kamin effect (Kamin, 1968). In the blocking paradigm, a previously neutral stimulus S_1 is conditioned to elicit a startle response (Phase I). During Phase II, a second stimulus S_2 is added to S_1 to form a compound stimulus while startle conditioning continues. The test condition (Phase III) involves presentation of S_2 alone to determine if it elicits the conditioned startle response. Socially reared monkeys exhibited the expected blocking. That is, they exhibited few, if any, startle responses to S_2. In contrast, socially isolated monkeys completely failed to exhibit blocking. This associative task demonstrated that in control monkeys the conditioning of a stimulus S_2 to elicit a startle response could be blocked if it was paired with S_1, a stimulus previously conditioned to elicit a startle response. Blocking has been demonstrated many times and is thought to be due to the fact that control subjects do not attend to S_2 as it provides no new information. Socially deprived monkeys, however, completely failed to exhibit blocking, a finding that suggests they are unable to ignore irrelevant or redundant information.

Central dopamine function has been shown to mediate, at least in part, the blocking phenomenon. For example, chronic d-amphetamine administration has been shown to disrupt blocking, an effect that can be restored with haloperidol (Crider, Solomon, & McMahon, 1982). Moreover, inducing dopamine receptor supersensitivity by chronic antagonist treatment also markedly attenuates blocking (Crider, Blockel, & Solomon, 1986). Jones, Gray, and Hensley (1992) reported the loss of the Kamin blocking effect in persons with acute schizophrenia. Similar studies have also established an important role for dopamine in the mediation of similar sensory-gating tasks such as latent inhibition and prepulse inhibition (inhibition of startle by presentation of a weak stimulus immediately preceding the more intense test stimulus). Thus, the blocking study provided the albeit indirectly, data to support the hypothesis of altered central dopamine function in socially deprived monkeys exhibiting high levels of stereotyped behavior.

CSF Monoamine Metabolites

One method of testing our hypothesis that dopamine or other monoamine systems were significantly altered by early social deprivation was to assay monoamine metabolites from the cerebrospinal fluid (CSF) of socially deprived and control monkeys. Cisternal CSF concentrations of homovanillic acid (HVA), 3-methoxy-4-hydroxyphenylethylene glycol (MHPG), and 5-hydroxyindoleacetic acid (5-HIAA), major metabolites of dopamine, norepinephrine, and serotonin, respectively, were found not to discriminate socially isolated from socially reared monkeys (Lewis, Gluck, Beauchamp, Keresztury, & Mailman, 1990). Thus, it would not appear that stereotyped behavior, at least in this model, is associated with major alterations in the release and metabolism of monoamine neurotransmitters. It should be remembered, however, that these measurements were done under basal conditions. Such data should be interpreted with caution because such measurements are likely to be responsive only to profound challenge. It may be that an environmental or pharmacologic challenge would have yielded rearing condition differences. Kraemer, Ebert, Lake, and McKinney (1983) reported rearing effects in the level of CSF norepinephrine in response to amphetamine challenge, a finding that supports this suggestion.

Dopamine Receptor Sensitivity

The hypothesis that stereotypy induced by early social deprivation is associated with alterations in dopamine receptor sensitivity subsequent to loss of presynaptic innervation was tested using older adult rhesus monkeys (Lewis et al., 1990). Both isolate and control monkeys were challenged with the direct-acting agonist apomorphine (0.1 and 0.3 mg/kg). The drug effects on spontaneous blink rate, stereotyped behavior, and self-injurious behavior were quantified using highly reliable observational measures. If, indeed, early isolation induces dopamine receptor supersensitivity, isolate monkeys should show a potentiated response to the drug. At the higher dose, apomorphine significantly increased the rate of spontaneous blinking; indeed, this behavior appeared to be the most sensitive to the developmental insult. Analysis of videotaped sequences of behavior showed that the occurrence of whole body, but not oral, stereotypies, as well as the intensity of stereotyped behavior (as measured by observer ratings), were significantly potentiated in isolate monkeys. The frequency of occurrence of self-injurious behavior was too low to allow for meaningful comparisons. These significant differences in response to apomorphine challenge support the hypothesis that long-term or permanent alterations in dopamine receptor sensitivity, as assessed by drug challenge, are a consequence of early social deprivation.

Functional Alterations in Brain

We have directly examined brain tissue from socially deprived and control monkeys using immunocytochemical techniques to visualize specific types of neurons (Martin, Spicer, Lewis, Gluck, & Cork, 1991). Early social deprivation profoundly affected the chemoarchitecture of the corpus striatum, the terminal field of the major dopamine projection in brain. Striatal tissue was processed immunocytochemically for tyrosine hydroxylase, a marker for dopamine neurons, as well as for substance P, leu-enkephalin, and somatostatin; neurons for these chemical messengers are found in abundance in striatal areas. Fibers, terminals, and cell bodies immunoreactive for substance P and leu-enkephalin were reduced in striata of socially deprived monkeys. Tyrosine hydroxylase immunoreactivity associated with terminals and fibers was also significantly reduced in the striatum of socially deprived animals. This indicates that dopamine innervation of this region is substantially reduced. Tyrosine hydroxylase staining was also markedly reduced (ca. 43%) in substantia nigra. These data indicate that early social deprivation substantially altered the innervation of the striatum by dopamine neurons. These results supported our initial hypotheses concerning the relationship of altered dopaminergic activity within the striatum and behavioral disturbances characteristic of the isolation syndrome. These results also complement the psychopharmacologic study with apomorphine. In the face of altered dopamine innervation, a consequent receptor supersensitivity might be expected to emerge.

Dopamine Receptor Changes

Functional supersensitivity of specific receptor types in response to denervation or disuse has historically been thought to be mediated by an increased receptor density. In order to characterize receptor alterations induced by early social deprivation and associated with stereotyped behavior, we used receptor autoradiographic techniques. Tissue sections at the level of striatum from both socially reared and socially deprived monkeys were labelled with ^{3}H-SCH23982 and ^{125}I-epidepride to quantify D_1 and D_2 binding sites, respectively. No effects of differential early experience on dopamine receptor density were apparent. This result is, in some ways, not surprising, as our work with rodent denervation models has shown that a profound functional supersensitivity can be obtained without an increased density of dopamine receptors (Mileson et al., 1991).

STEREOTYPED BEHAVIOR IN INDIVIDUALS WITH MENTAL RETARDATION

Stereotyped behavior in individuals with mental retardation has been the subject of a great deal of theoretical and empirical treatment (Baumeister & Forehand, 1973; Berkson, 1967; Lewis & Baumeister, 1982). The most frequently observed behavioral categories falling under this rubric include body rocking, head rolling, and repetitive hand movements. Baumeister and Forehand estimated that these behaviors occur in two-thirds of the population institutionalized for mental retardation. Stereotypies interfere with habilitative efforts and the expression of socially adaptive behavior. Stereotyped behavior also includes certain forms of self-injurious behavior that result in acute physical damage to the individual. Self-hitting, head banging, and self-biting are among the most common topographies of self-injury (Baumeister & Rollings, 1976). These behaviors represent a major management problem for clinical staff, pose a threat to the safety of the individual, and are often difficult to suppress over time and across various settings. To our knowledge, there has been no *systematic* research aimed at elucidating the neurobiological basis of stereotyped behavior in persons with mental retardation. This is despite the high prevalence of stereotypies in this group and the fact that such behavior often dominates the repertoire of the individual.

Spontaneous Blink Rates and Stereotypies: Evidence for Dopamine Involvement

Evidence for the predominant role played by dopamine in mediating spontaneous blink rate comes from research involving persons with schizophrenia and Parkinson's disease, as well as from studies of nonhuman primates (Karson, 1983; Karson, Staub, Kleinman, & Wyatt, 1981). Significantly decreased blink rates were reported as early as the 1920s in persons with Parkinson's disease. Subsequent studies have demonstrated that dopamine agonists increase blink rates in both humans and non-human primates, whereas dopamine antagonists reduce spontaneous blinking. Our work suggested that spontaneous blink rate in nonhuman primates may be among the most sensitive behavioral indices of dopamine receptor activation, particularly in dopamine-depleted animals (Elsworth et al., 1991; Lewis et al., 1990).

We compared the spontaneous blink rates of persons with mental retardation who engaged in high rates of stereotyped behavior with matched control participants (MacLean, Lewis, Bryson-Brockman, Ellis, Arendt, & Baumeister, 1985). In that study, eye blink rates were recorded during periods of both stereotyped and nonstereotyped behavior. Men, but not women, who engaged in stereotypy exhibited significantly lower blink rates than did the men who participated as control subjects. The low blink rates observed in women participants, particularly the control group, were correlated with the presence of irregular menstrual cycles or amenorrhea. Additionally, blink rate was found to be inversely correlated with the percent time engaged in stereotypy. Interestingly, no significant difference in blinking was observed between periods of stereotyped activity versus periods during which no stereotyped behavior occurred. The significantly lower rates of spontaneous blinking observed in male stereotypy participants versus same-sex control participants suggested decreased dopaminergic activity and, possibly, dopamine receptor supersensitivity. Indeed, the rates observed in male stereotypy participants were comparable to the blink rates reported for individuals with advanced Parkinson's disease (Karson, LeWitt, Calne, & Wyatt, 1982). The women who acted as control subjects were found to have significantly lower blink rates than those of their male counterparts. They also had somewhat lower blink rates than did the women with stereotypies. The low blink rate observed in the latter group appeared to be related to the higher percentage of amenorrheic participants. This finding suggested that gonadal steroids, particularly estrogen, determine, at least in part, blink rate. This is consistent with the underlying hypothesis of the present work because there is ample evidence in the literature that indicates estrogen modulates dopamine function, including dopamine receptor sensitivity. This may well explain the gender differences observed here (e.g., Joyce, Montero, & Vantartesveldt, 1984).

We recently replicated the findings of the MacLean et al. (1985) study (Bodfish, Powell, Golden, & Lewis, 1995). Participants in the recent study had received antipsychotic medication for at least 1 year before the initiation of the study. Blink rates for the two groups were observed across five different daily sessions. The data allowed us to demonstrate the stability or reliability of this measure when quantified in a controlled setting. Statistical analysis of group differences showed significantly lower blink rates in stereotypy participants versus matched control participants. Moreover, significant inverse correlations were found for blink rate and severity of repetitive behavior disorder, and for blink rate and ratings of motor slowness. These data further support our hypothesis of decreased dopamine and provide an important replication of our earlier work.

In our work with vervet monkeys, we demonstrated that eye blink rate is mediated by both D_1 and D_2 receptors; activation of either receptor subtype with a selective agonist increased blink rate (Elsworth et al., 1991). Further, selective antagonists blocked only the blinking induced by agonists selective for the same receptor subtype. These data suggest that these dopamine receptor subtypes function independently in mediating blinking.

Psychopharmacology of Stereotyped Behavior in Mentally Retarded People

Hypotheses concerning the neurobiological basis of clinical disorders often are based on serendipitous observations of the efficacy of certain treatments. If the mechanism of action of the successful therapy can be established, then hypotheses can be made about the pathophysiology of the disorder. In the case of pathological stereotypies, pharmacologic interventions of proven efficacy are largely lacking. The mainstay of pharmacotherapy for persons with mental retardation has been antipsychotic drugs. It is estimated that almost 50% of the people with mental retardation living in residential facilities, and more than 20% of those who reside in the community are receiving antipsychotic drugs (Hill, Balow, & Bruininks, 1985; Intagliata & Rinck, 1985). Chadsey-Rusch and Sprague (1989) reported that individuals perceived to engage in stereotyped behavior tended to be kept on such medication despite a lack of compelling evidence for the efficacy of such treatment. Moreover, this class of drugs may increase the risk of long-term neurological side effects such as tardive dyskinesia and may have detrimental effects on learning and performance.

Several studies have supported the utility of antipsychotic drugs (see Baumeister & Sevin, 1990, for a review); however, in some cases, only modest treatment effects have been reported (e.g., Aman, White, & Field, 1984). Still other studies have demonstrated either a lack of efficacy for antipsychotic drugs or an exacerbation of stereotyped behavior associated with such treatment (Heistad, Zimmermann, & Doebler, 1982; Lewis et al., 1986). Indeed, our own work with thioridazine suggests not only that this drug is ineffective in controlling stereotypies, but also that drug administration *exacerbates* stereotyped responding in a significant number of persons (Lewis et al.). This result may relate to the potent anticholinergic effects of thioridazine. In any case, there are clearly many examples of individuals displaying high rates of stereotyped behavior while they are being treated with high doses of antipsychotic drugs. Thus, the conclusion that antipsychotic drugs are effective in treating the stereotyped behavior associated with mental retardation is, at best, premature and may be unwarranted. Explicit note must be made, however, of recent advances in understanding the function of multiple dopamine receptors. It well may be that receptor subtype–selective antagonists might yet be of utility, although this is purely speculative.

The only other class of drugs that has been systematically examined for its effects against stereotyped behavior is that of the opiate antagonists. Whereas positive effects have been reported with regard to self-injurious behavior, naltrexone was not found to be effective in suppressing stereotyped behavior in persons with mental retardation (Sandman, Barron, & Coleman, 1990), although more recent evidence may provide some support for its efficacy.

Stereotyped and Compulsive Behavior

Dantzer (1986) defined stereotypy as "repetitive sequences of activities that consist of a few fixed elements carried out at a higher than normal rate and occurring in nearly the same order in successive cycles" (p. 1777). This characterization is strikingly similar to the definition of compulsions provided by the American Psychiatric Association's (1987) *Diagnostic and Statistical Manual*. The most common compulsions involve hand washing, counting, checking, and touching (Rapoport, 1989).

Studies of obsessive–compulsive disorder (OCD) have direct relevance to the present discussion, specifically as they relate to involuntary motor movements. For example, approximately 20% of patients with OCD display motor tics (Rapoport, 1989). Indeed, OCD is known to occur in conjunction with diseases of the basal ganglia, including Syndenham's chorea, postencephalitic Parkinson's disease, Tourette's syndrome, and toxic lesions of the striatum (Rapoport, 1988). Obsessive–compulsive behavior and self-injurious behavior are frequently co-expressed (Primeau & Fontaine, 1987), particularly in patients with Tourette's syndrome (Trimble, 1989). It has been hypothesized that, because the basal ganglia play a fundamental role in sensory–motor integration, perturbations in this brain region may result in a disinhibition of behavioral output. Several recent in vivo imaging studies conducted with patients with OCD supported the hypothesis of basal ganglia dysfunction. These results included increased caudate nucleus volume as determined by computed axial tomography (CAT) scans and increased glucose metabolism in the frontal lobe, cingulate pathway, and caudate nucleus (Swedo, Shapiro et al., 1989; Swedo, Leonard, et al., 1989). These observations are particularly relevant as numerous animal studies, some of which have been described in this chapter, have demonstrated the importance of the basal ganglia in the mediation of stereotyped behavior.

It is also important to note the ethological perspective adopted by several investigators studying OCD. Compulsive, ritualistic behaviors in humans are similar to the fixed action patterns described by animal behaviorists (Pitman, 1989; Rapoport, 1989). Studies have also focused on similar animal paradigms such as displacement activities, schedule-induced behavior, and lateral hypothalamic stimulation (e.g., Pitman, 1989) as potentially useful animal models. As we argued earlier (Lewis & Baumeister, 1982) stereotyped behavior seen in persons with mental retardation should not be viewed as a self-contained category of aberrant behavior. Rather, its similarities to behavioral phenomena such as displacement activity, schedule-induced behavior, and stimulant-induced motor activity should be recognized and integrated into theories of the biological basis and function of such behavior. Thus, compulsive/ritualistic behavior, stereotyped behavior, and the other behavioral models described appear to share important similarities, perhaps including common neurobiological substrates. In this regard, striatal serotonin–dopamine interactions appear to be particularly important candidates for study.

Stereotypies and Compulsive Behavior Disorder: Comorbidity

Our group has found direct evidence to support the hypothesis that stereotyped behavior is comorbid in individuals with mental retardation who display compulsive behavior disorder (Bodfish, Crawford et al., 1995; Crawford & Bodfish, 1992). In our sample, 59% were identified as having motor stereotypies, 48.7% were identified as having self-injury, and 38.5% were identified as having compulsive/ritualistic behaviors. Interestingly, the occurrence of compulsive behavior disorder was associated with an increased prevalence of stereotypy of 32%, an increased prevalence of self-injury of 40%, and an increased prevalence of both stereotypy and self-injury of 37% compared with a noncompulsive matched control group.

Because an abnormal growth rate has been observed in patients with OCD, we examined physical stature in individuals with mental retardation who displayed repetitive movement disorders (Powell, Bodfish, Crawford, Golden, & Lewis, in press). Women with mental retardation and compulsive behavior disorder—but not stereotyped movement disorder—were significantly shorter and weighed significantly less than their control counterparts. Conversely, men with stereotyped movement disorder—but not compulsive disorder—were significantly shorter and weighed significantly less than same sex-control participants. These findings may point to a neuroendocrine abnormality associated with repetitive movement disorders such as stereotypy.

Alterations in serotonergic function have been most frequently linked with OCD, and the treatment of choice for this disorder has been antidepressant medications that selectively inhibit the uptake of serotonin. Thus, we examined the efficacy of the serotonin uptake inhibitor fluoxetine in the treatment of compulsions (Bodfish & Madison, 1993). Using a group comparison, prepost open-trial methodology, we found that treatment with fluoxetine resulted in a significant decrease in aggression and self-injury in a compulsive behavior disorder group, but not in matched noncompulsive control participants. Interestingly, a relationship did exist among stereotypies, compulsions, and fluoxetine response. A majority (70%) of the compulsive fluoxetine responders displayed stereotypies, whereas only a few (17%) of the noncompulsive, and fluoxetine nonresponders did so. A similar relation was found for self-injury, compulsion, and fluoxetine response.

The similarity between stereotyped behavior and OCD provided a strong rationale for evaluating systematically the potential efficacy of antidepressant drugs in the treatment of stereotypies. We examined the efficacy of the serotonin (5-HT) uptake inhibitor clomipramine in the treatment of stereotyped and related repetitive behavior disorders in individuals with severe and profound mental retardation (Lewis, Bodfish, Powell, & Golden, 1995). Significant reductions in the frequency and intensity of stereotyped behavior, teacher ratings of stereotypy, increased adaptive engagement, and decreased staff intervention for nontargeted behavior problems were all observed following the administration of clomipramine. These results provided support for the hypothesis that clomipramine may be efficacious in the treatment of stereotyped and related behavior. The study also represented the first controlled trial of a 5-HT uptake inhibitor in the treatment of repetitive behavior disorders in mental retardation.

CONCLUSION

We have focused on three different models of stereotyped behavior: drug-induced stereotypies in rodents, abnormal stereotypies in rhesus monkeys induced by early social deprivation, and stereotyped movement disorder observed so frequently in individuals with severe mental retardation. The results reviewed here highlight the importance of striatal dopamine in the mediation of stereotyped behavior in all three models. One central question still to be resolved is what the specific alterations are in dopamine function that result in the expression of stereotyped behavior in clinical disorders such as severe retardation and autism. A corollary to this is whether such changes are secondary to other neural perturbations. Other neurotransmitters or neuromodulators (e.g., serotonin) must assuredly play an important role in the expression of this complex behavior. Our findings have generally supported the hypothesis that stereotyped movement disorder is associated with impaired dopamine function, involving decreased synaptic concentrations of dopamine with subsequent increased sensitivity of dopamine receptors. The basis for this hypothesis comes from several observations made by our group. The first involved the significantly increased likelihood of stereotyped responding following pharmacologic challenge in dopamine-depleted rats. The second observation involved the potentiated response (i.e., greater stereotyped behavior) to the dopamine agonist apomorphine in socially deprived monkeys. Such behavioral supersensitivity usually is a consequence of decreases in the synaptic availability of dopamine. The third observation involved the substantial reduction of tyrosine hydroxylase immunoreactivity (a marker for dopamine neurons) in the striatum and substantia nigra of socially deprived reared monkeys. The final observation involved the significantly decreased blink rates observed in men with mental retardation who had a history of stereotyped behavior.

What are the implications of these findings for pharmacotherapy? As already noted, there has been little systematic effort to examine the efficacy of various classes of psychotropic drugs in the treatment of stereotyped movement disorder. Data on the effectiveness of antipsychotics are ambiguous, and some other drug classes such as opiate antagonists do not appear particularly promising. We have initiated studies examining the efficacy of 5-HT uptake inhibitors in treating stereotypies based on the similarities of OCD to stereotyped movement disorder and evidence for their comorbidity. We believe these compounds are promising. Finally, if striatal dopamine depletion is a key element of the pathophysiology of stereotyped movement disorder, then long-term treatment with antipsychotic drugs may be deleterious. In the short run, antipsychotics may mask some of the behavioral symptoms associated with dopamine receptor supersensitivity, but prolonged blockade of such receptors may well augment the effects of dopamine depletion. These concerns, as well as concerns with the questionable efficacy and deleterious adverse effects of antipsychotics, should be important considerations in clinical treatment decisions. Conversely, the use of compounds that act in brain to increase synaptic concentrations of dopamine or directly activate dopamine receptors may prove useful. Carefully controlled clinical trials based on rational pharmacotherapy are badly needed.

It is clear that considerably more work will be required before we can make any conclusive statements about the neurobiological basis of stereotyped movement disorder. Various hypotheses need to be tested rigorously by means of multiple methodologies. Some of these hypotheses concerning alterations in specific neurotransmitter systems can be tested in vivo using neuroendocrine challenge paradigms. Such approaches, used frequently in biological psychiatry, involve the intravenous infusion of a drug that has selective effects on a class of neurotransmitter receptors. Differential effects of the drug–receptor interaction can then be assessed by measuring endocrine changes mediated by that class of receptor. This strategy is useful if there is a hormone response linked to the same receptor population(s) believed to be involved in the behavior under study.

A second avenue for studying the neurobiology of stereotypies is the use of increasingly sophisticated neuroimaging technologies. Cerebral blood flow, structural alterations in specific brain areas, neuronal activity as measured by glucose uptake, and the density of certain classes of neurotransmitter receptors can all be measured in the living organism. More and better controlled clinical trials of drugs that have reasonably selective effects in the CNS would be a substantial contribution not only to the development of better therapies, but also to a better understanding of the pathophysiology of stereotyped movement disorder. Continued study of a variety of animal models of stereotyped behavior is critical. Such studies represent a rich source of information, as stereotypies can be observed in animals under a variety of experimental conditions. Finally, detailed examination of postmortem material promises to provide perhaps the least ambiguous way to assess alterations in CNS that accompany stereotyped movement disorder.

The study of stereotyped behavior can provide a wealth of information about brain–behavior relationships and the behavioral consequences of brain insult. A fundamental question to pursue is why stereotyped behavior appears to be such a frequent behavioral outcome of a wide variety of perturbations that alter CNS activity. These and other fundamental questions in the study of stereotypy await answers.

REFERENCES

Aman, M. G., White, A. J., & Field, C. (1984). Chlorpromazine effects on stereotypic and conditioned behaviour of severely retarded patients—A pilot study. *Journal of Mental Deficiency Research, 28,* 253–260.

American Psychiatric Association. (1987). *Diagnostic and statistical manual of mental disorders (3rd.-rev.),* Washington, DC: Author.

Anderson, J., Gingrich, J., Bates, M., Dearry, A., Faladeau, P., Senogles, S., & Caron, M. (1990). Dopamine receptor subtypes: Beyond the D1/D2 classification. *Trends in Pharmacological Sciences, 22,* 231–236.

Arnt, J., Hyttel, J., & Perregard, J. (1987). Dopamine D-1 receptor agonists combined with the selective D-2 agonist quinpirole facilitate the expression of oral stereotyped behavior in rats. *European Journal of Pharmacology, 133,* 137–145.

Baumeister, A. A., & Forehand, R. (1973). Stereotyped acts. In N. R. Ellis (Ed.), *International review of research in mental retardation* (Vol. 6, pp. 55–96). New York: Academic Press.

Baumeister, A. A., & Rollings, J. P. (1976). Self-injurious behavior. In N. R. Ellis (Ed.), *International review of research in mental retardation* (Vol. 8, pp. 1–34). New York: Academic Press.

Baumeister, A. A., & Sevin, J. A. (1990). Pharmacologic control of aberrant behavior in the mentally retarded: Toward a more rational approach. *Neuroscience and Biobehavioral Reviews, 14,* 253–262.

Beauchamp, A. J., Gluck, J. P., & Lewis, M. H. (1991). Associative processes in differentially reared rhesus monkeys (*Macaca mulatta*): Blocking. *Developmental Psychobiology, 24,* 175–189.

Berkson, G. (1967). Abnormal stereotyped motor acts. In J. Zubin & H. F. Hunt (Eds.), *Comparative psychopathology: Animal and human* (76–94). New York: Grune & Stratton.

Berkson, G. (1983). Repetitive stereotyped behaviors. *American Journal of Mental Deficiency, 88,* 239–246.

Bodfish, J. W., Crawford, T. W., Powell, S. B., Parker, D. E., Golden, R. N., & Lewis, M. H. (1995). Compulsions in adults with mental retardation: Prevalence, phenomenology, and comorbidity with stereotypy and self-injury. *American Journal of Mental Retardation, 100,* 183–192.

Bodfish, J. W., & Madison, J. T. (1993). Diagnosis and fluoxetine treatment of compulsive behavior disorder of adults with mental retardation. *American Journal of Mental Retardation, 98,* 360–367.

Bodfish, J. W., Powell, S. B., Golden, R. N., Lewis, M. H. (1995). Blink rate as an index of dopamine function in adults with mental retardation and repetitive behavior disorders. *American Journal of Mental Retardation, 99,* 335–344.

Bordi, F., & Meller, E. (1989). Enhanced behavioral stereotypies elicited by intrastriatal injection of D_1 and D_2 dopamine agonists in intact rats. *Brain Research, 504,* 276–283.

Braun, A. R., & Chase, T. N. (1986). Obligatory D-1/D-2 receptor interaction in the generation of dopamine agonist related behaviors. *European Journal of Pharmacology, 131,* 301–306.

Brett, L. P., & Levine, S. (1979). Schedule-induced polydipsia and pituitary–adrenal activity in rats. *Journal of Comparative and Physiological Psychology, 93,* 946–956.

Brewster, W. K., Nichols, D. E., Riggs, R. M., Mottola, D. M., Lovenberg, T. W., Lewis, M. H., & Mailman, R. B. (1990). Trans-10,11-dihydroxy-5,6,6a,7,8,12b-hexahydrobenzo[a]-phenanthridine: A highly potent selective dopamine D_1 full agonist. *Journal of Medicinal Chemistry, 33,* 1756–1764.

Chadsey-Rusch, J., & Sprague, R. L. (1989). Maladaptive behaviors associated with neuroleptic drug maintenance. *American Journal of Mental Retardation, 93,* 607–617.

Clark, D., & White, F. J. (1987). D_1 dopamine receptor—The search for a function. A critical evaluation of the D_1/D_2 dopamine receptor classification and its functional implications. *Synapse, 1,* 347–388.

Cooper, S. J., & Dourish, C. T. (1990). Historical perspectives on dopamine and stereotypy. In S. J. Cooper & C. T. Dourish (Eds.), *Neurobiology of stereotyped behaviour* (pp. 1–24). Oxford, England: Oxford University Press.

Crawford, T. W., & Bodfish, J. W. (1992). Obsessive–compulsive disorder. In E. A. Konarski, J. E. Favell, & J. E. Favell (Eds.), *Manual for the assessment and treatment of the behavior disorders of people with mental retardation* (pp. 1–13). Morganton, NC: Western Carolina Center Foundation.

Creese, I., & Iversen, S. D. (1973). Blockage of amphetamine-induced motor stimulation and stereotypy in the adult rat following neonatal treatment with 6-hydroxydopamine. *Brain Research, 55,* 369–382.

Creese, I., Sibley, D. R., Hamblin, M. W., & Leff, S. E. (1983). The classification of dopamine receptors: Relationship to radioligand binding. *Annual Review of Neuroscience, 6,* 43–71.

Crider, A., Blockel, L., & Solomon, P. R. (1986). A selective attention deficit in the rat following induced dopamine receptor supersensitivity. *Behavioral Neuroscience, 100,* 315–319.

Crider, A., Solomon, P. R., & McMahon, M. (1982). Disruption of attention in the rat following chronic d-amphetamine administration: Possible relation to schizophrenic attention disorder. *Biological Psychiatry, 17,* 351–361.

Curzon, G. (1990). Stereotyped and other motor responses to 5-hydroxytryptamine receptor activation. In S. J. Cooper & C. T. Dourish (Eds.), *Neurobiology of stereotyped behaviour* (pp. 142–168). Oxford, England: Oxford University Press.

Dantzer, R. (1986). Behavioral, physiological and functional aspects of stereotyped behavior: A review and re-interpretation. *Journal of Animal Science, 62,* 1776–1786.

Darney, K. J., Jr., Lewis, M. H., Brewster, W. K., Nichols, D. E., & Mailman, R. B. (1991). Behavioral effects in the rat of dihydrexidine, a high potency, full efficacy D_1 dopamine receptor agonist. *Neuropsychopharmacology, 5,* 187–195.

Duncan, I. J. H., & Wood-Gush, D. G. M. (1972). Thwarting of feeding behavior in the domestic fowl. *Animal Behaviour, 20,* 444–451.

Ellinwood, E. H., Jr. (1967). Amphetamine psychosis: I. Description of the individuals and process. *Journal of Nervous and Mental Disease, 144,* 273–282.

Ellinwood, E. H., Jr. (1969). Amphetamine psychosis: A multi-dimensional process. *Seminars in Psychiatry, 1,* 208–226.

Elsworth, J. D., Lawrence, M. S., Roth, R. H., Taylor, J. R., Mailman, R. B., Nichols, D. E., Lewis, M. H., & Redmond, D. E., Jr. (1991). D_1 and D_2 dopamine receptors independently regulate spontaneous blink rate in the vervet monkey. *Journal of Pharmacology and Experimental Therapeutics, 259,* 595–600.

Ernst, A. M., & Smelik, P. G. (1966). Site of action of dopamine and apomorphine on compulsive gnawing behavior in rats. *Experientia, 22,* 837–838.

Fentress, J. C. (1976). Dynamic boundaries of patterned behaviors: Interaction and self-organization. In P. P. G. Bateson & R. A. Hinde (Eds.), *Growing points in ethology* (pp. 135–169). London: Cambridge University Press.

Ferre, S., Von Euler, G., Johansson, B., Fredholm, B., & Fuxe, K. (1991). Stimulation of high affinity adenosine A-2 receptors decreases the affinity of dopamine D-2 receptors in rat striatal membranes. *Proceedings of the National Academy of Sciences, 88,* 7238–7241.

Fog, R. (1972). On the stereotypy and catalepsy studies on the effect of amphetamines and neuroleptics in rats. *Acta Neurologica Scandanavica, 38* (Suppl. 500), 11–66.

Garau, L., Govoni, S., Stefanini, E., Trabucchi, M., & Spano, P. F. (1978). Dopamine receptors: Pharmacological and anatomical evidences indicate that two distinct dopamine receptor populations are present in rat striatum. *Life Sciences, 23,* 1745–1750.

Goosen, C. (1981) Abnormal behavior patterns in rhesus monkeys: Symptoms of mental disease? *Biological Psychiatry, 16,* 697–716.

Harlow, H. F., Dodsworth, R. O., & Harlow, M. K. (1965). Total social isolation in monkeys. *Proceedings of the National Academy of Sciences, 54,* 90–97.

Heistad, G. T., Zimmermann, R. L., & Doebler, M. I. (1982). Long-term usefulness of thioridazine for institutionalized mentally retarded patients. *American Journal of Mental Deficiency, 87,* 243–251.

Hill, B. K., Balow, E. A., & Bruininks, R. H. (1985). A national study of prescribed drugs in institutions and community residential facilities for mentally retarded people. *Psychopharmacology Bulletin, 21,* 279–284.

Hutt, C., Hutt, S. J., Lee, D., & Ousted, C. (1964). Arousal and childhood autism. *Nature, 204,* 908–909.

Intagliata, J., & Rinck, C. (1985). Psychoactive drug use in public and community residential facilities for mentally retarded persons. *Psychopharmacology Bulletin, 21,* 268–278.

Isaacson, R. L., & Gispen, W. H. (1990). Neuropeptides and the issue of stereotypy in behaviour. In S. J. Cooper & C. T. Dourish (Eds.), *Neurobiology of stereotyped behaviour.* Oxford, England: Oxford University Press.

Iwamoto, E. T., & Way, E. L. (1977). Circling behavior and stereotypy induced by intranigral opiate microinjection. *Journal of Pharmacology and Experimental Therapeutics, 20,* 347–359.

Janssen, P. A. J., Niemegeers, C. J. E., & Schellekens, K. H. L. (1965). Is it possible to predict the clinical effects of neuroleptic drugs (major tranquilizers) from animal data? (Part I). *Arzneimittel-Forschung, 15,* 104–117.

Janssen, P. A. J., Niemegeers, C. J. E., Schellekens, K. H. L., & Leanerts, F. M. (1967). Is it possible to predict the clinical effects of neuroleptic drugs (major tranquilizers) from animal data? (Part IV). *Arzneimittel-Forschung, 17,* 841–854.

Jones, S. H., Gray, J. A., & Hensley, D. R. (1992). Loss of the Kamin blocking effect in acute but not chronic schizophrenics. *Biological Psychiatry, 32,* 739–755.

Joyce, J. N., Montero, E., & Van Hartesveldt, C. (1984). Dopamine-mediated behaviors: Characteristics of modulation by estrogen. *Pharmacology, Biochemistry and Behavior, 21,* 791–800.

Kamin, L. J. (1968). Attention-like processes in classical conditioning. In M. R. Jones (Ed.), *Miami symposium on the prediction of behavior: Aversive stimulation.* Miami: University of Miami Press.

Karson, C. N. (1983). Spontaneous eye-blink rates and dopaminergic systems. *Brain, 106,* 643–653.

Karson, C. N., LeWitt, P. A., Calne, D. B., & Wyatt, R. J. (1982). Blink rates in Parkinsonism. *Annals of Neurology, 12,* 580–583.

Karson, C. N., Staub, R. A., Kleinman, J. E., & Wyatt, R. J. (1981). Drug effect on blink rates in rhesus monkeys: Preliminary studies. *Biological Psychiatry, 16,* 249–254.

Kebabian, J. W., & Calne, D. B. (1979). Multiple receptors for dopamine. *Nature, 277,* 93–96.

Kraemer, G. W., Ebert, M. H., Lake, C. R., & McKinney, W. T. (1983). Amphetamine challenge: Effects in previously isolated rhesus monkeys and implications for animal models of schizophrenia. In K. A. Miczek (Ed.), *Ethopharmacology: Primate models of neuropsychiatric disorders.* New York: A. R. Liss.

Kulik, A. V., & Wilbur, R. (1982). Delirium and stereotypy from anticholinergic antiparkinson drugs. *Progress in Neuropsychopharmacology and Biological Psychiatry, 6,* 75–82.

Levy, D. M. (1944). On the problem of movement restraint. *American Journal of Orthopsychiatry, 14,* 644–677.

Lewis, M. H., & Baumeister, A. A. (1982). Stereotyped mannerisms in mentally retarded persons: Animal models and theoretical analyses. In N. R. Ellis (Ed.), *In-*

ternational review of research in mental retardation (Vol. 11, 123–161). New York: Academic Press.

Lewis, M. H., Baumeister, A. A., & Mailman, R. B. (1987). A neurobiological alternative to the perceptual reinforcement hypothesis of stereotyped behavior: A commentary on "self-stimulatory behavior and perceptual reinforcement." *Journal of Applied Behavior Analysis, 20,* 253–258.

Lewis, M. H., Baumeister, A. A., McCorkle, D. L., & Mailman, R. B. (1985). A computer supported method for analyzing behavioral observations: Studies with stereotypy. *Psychopharmacology, 85,* 204–209.

Lewis, M. H., Bodfish, J. W., Powell, S. B., & Golden, R. N. (1995). Clomipramine treatment for stereotypy and related repetitive movement disorders associated with mental retardation. *American Journal of Mental Retardation, 100,* 299–312.

Lewis, M. H., Gluck, J. P., Beachamp, A. J., Keresztury, M. F., & Mailman, R. B. (1990). Long-term effects of early social isolation in *Macaca mulatta*: In vivo evidence for changes in dopamine receptor function. *Brain Research, 513,* 67–73.

Lewis, M. H., MacLean, W. E., Bryson-Brockman, W., Arendt, R., Beck, B., Fidler, P., & Baumeister, A. A. (1984). Time-series analysis of stereotyped movements: The relationship of body rocking to cardiac activity. *American Journal of Mental Deficiency, 89,* 287–294.

Lewis, M. H., Steer, R. A., Favell, J., McGimsey, J., Clontz, L., Trivette, C., Jodry, W., Schroeder, S., Kanoy, R., & Mailman, R. B. (1986). Thioridazine metabolism and effects on stereotyped behavior in mentally retarded patients. *Psychopharmacology Bulletin, 22,* 1040–1044.

Lovaas, O. I., Newsom, C., & Hickman, C. (1987). Self-stimulatory behavior and perceptual reinforcement. *Journal of Applied Behavior Analysis, 20,* 45–68.

Lovenberg, T. W., Brewster, W. K., Mottola, D. M., Lee, R. C., Riggs, R. M., Nichols, D. E., Lewis, M. H., & Mailman, R. B. (1989). Dihydrexidine, a novel selective high potency full dopamine D_1 receptor agonist. *European Journal of Pharmacology, 166,* 111–113.

MacLean, W. E., Jr., Lewis, M. H., Bryson-Brockmann, W. A., Ellis, D. N., Arendt, R. E., & Baumeister, A. A. (1985). Blink rate and stereotyped behavior: Evidence for dopamine involvement? *Biological Psychiatry, 20,* 1321–1325.

Mailman, R. B., Schulz, D. W., Lewis, M. H., Staples, L., Rollema, H., & Dehaven, D. L. (1984). SCH23390: A selective D_1 dopamine antagonist with potent D_2 behavioral actions. *European Journal of Pharmacology, 101,* 159–160.

Martin, L., Spicer, D. W., Lewis, M. H., Gluck, J. P., & Cork, L. C. (1991). Social deprivation in infant rhesus monkeys alters the chemoarchitecture of the brain: I. Subcortical regions. *Journal of Neuroscience, 11,* 3344–3358.

Mashurano, M., & Waddington, J. L. (1986). Stereotyped behavior in response to the selective D-2 dopamine receptor agonist RU24213 is enhanced by pretreatment with the selective D-1 agonist SK&F38393. *Neuropharmacology, 25,* 947–949.

Mason, G. (1991). Stereotypies: A critical review. *Animal Behaviour, 41,* 1015–1037.

Meller, E., Bordi, F., & Bohmaker, K. (1988). Enhancement by the D_1 dopamine agonist SKF38393 of specific components of stereotypy elicited by the D_2 agonists LY171555 and RU24213. *Life Sciences, 42,* 2561–2567.

Meyer-Holzapfel, M. (1968). Abnormal behaviour in zoo animals. In M. W. Fox (Ed.), *Abnormal behavior in animals.* London: Saunders.

Mileson, B. E., Lewis, M. H., & Mailman, R. B. (1991). Dopamine receptor supersensitivity occurring without receptor up-regulation. *Brain Research, 561,* 1–10.

Molloy, A. G., &Waddington, J. L. (1984). Dopaminergic behavior stereospecifically promoted by the D_1 agonist R-SK&F38393 and selectively blocked by the D_1 antagonist SCH23390. *Psychopharmacology, 82,* 409–410.

Mottola, D. M., Brewster, W. K., Cook, L. L., Nichols, D. E., & Mailman, R. B. (1992). Dihydrexidine, a novel full efficacy D_1 dopamine receptor agonist. *Journal of Pharmacology and Experimental Therapeutics, 262,* 383–393.

Pitman, R. K. (1989). Animal models of compulsive behavior. *Biological Psychiatry, 26,* 189–198.

Pope, S. G., Dean, P., & Redgrave, P. (1980). Dissociation of d-amphetamine induced locomotor activity and stereotyped behavior by lesions of the superior colliculus. *Psychopharmacology, 70,* 297–302.

Powell, S. B., Bodfish, J. W., Crawford, T. W., Golden, R. N., & Lewis, M. H. (in press). Growth differences associated with compulsive and stereotyped behavior disorders in adults with mental retardation. *J. Anxiety.*

Primeau, F., & Fontaine, R. (1987). Obsessive disorder with self-mutilation: A subgroup responsive to pharmacotherapy. *Canadian Journal of Psychiatry, 32,* 699–701.

Randrup, A., & Munkvad, I. (1967). Stereotyped activities produced by amphetamines in several animal species and men. *Psychopharmacology, 11,* 300–310.

Rapoport, J. L. (1988). The neurobiology of obsessive–compulsive disorder. *Journal of the American Psychological Association, 260,* 2888–2890.

Rapoport, J. L. (1989, March). The biology of obsessions and compulsions. *Scientific American,* pp. 83–89.

Redgrave, P., Dean, P., Donohoe, T. P., & Pope, S. P. (1980). Superior colliculus lesions selectively attenuate apomorphine-induced oral stereotypy: A possible role for the nigrotectal pathway. *Brain Research, 196,* 541–546.

Ridley, R. F., Baker, H. F., & Scraggs, P. R. (1979). The time course of the behavioral effects of amphetamine and their reversal by haloperidol in a primate species. *Biological Psychiatry, 14,* 753–765.

Ridley, R. M., & Baker, H. F. (1982). Stereotypy in monkeys and humans. *Psychological Medicine, 12,* 61–72.

Rylander, G. (1971). Stereotypy in man following amphetamine abuse. In S. B. de Baker (Ed.), *The correlation of adverse effects in man with observations in animals* (pp. 29–31). Amsterdam: Excerpta Medica (International Congress Series No. 220).

Sandman, C. A., Barron, J. L., Chicz-DeMet, A., & DeMet, E. (1990). Plasma β-endorphin levels in patients with self-injurious behavior and stereotypy. *American Journal of Mental Retardation, 95,* 84–92.

Sandman, C. A., Barron, J. L., & Coleman, H. (1990). An orally administered opiate blocker, naltrexone, attenuates self-injurious behavior. *American Journal of Mental Retardation, 95,* 93–102.

Scheel-Kruger, J., Arnt, J., Braestrup, C., Christensen, A. V., Cools, A. R., & Magelund, G. (1978). GABA-dopamine interactions in substantia nigra and nucleus accumbens—Relevance to behavioral stimulation and stereotyped behavior. In P. J. Roberts, G. N. Woodruff, & L. L. Iversen (Eds.), *Advances in biochemical psychopharmacology* (Vol. 19, pp. 343–346). New York: Raven.

Scheel-Kruger, J., Arnt, J., Magelund, G., Olianas, M., Przewlocka, B., & Christensen, A. V. (1980). Behavioral functions of GABA in basal ganglia and limbic system. *Brain Research Bulletin, 5,* 261–267.

Swedo, S., Leonard, H., Rapoport, J., Lenane, M. C., Goldberger, E. L., & Cheslow, D. L. (1989). A double-blind comparison of clomipramine and desipramine in the treatment of trichotillomania (hair pulling). *New England Journal of Medicine, 321,* 497–501.

Swedo, S. E., Schapiro, M. B., Grady, C. L., Cheslow, D. L., Leonard, H. L., Kumar, A., Friedland, R., Rapoport, S. I., & Rapoport, J. L. (1989). Cerebral glucose metabolism in childhood-onset obsessive–compulsive disorder. *Archives of General Psychiatry, 46,* 518–523.

Thelen, E. (1981). Rhythmical behavior in infancy: An ethological perspective. *Developmental Psychology, 17,* 237–257.

Trimble, M. (1989). Psychopathology and movement disorders: A new perspective on the Gilles de la Tourette syndrome. *Journal of Neurology, Neurosurgery, and Psychiatry* Suppl (Jun), 90–95.

Ungerstedt, U. (1971). Postsynaptic supersensitivity after 6-hydroxydopamine induced degeneration of the nigro-striatal dopamine system. *Acta Physiologica Scandinavica, 367*, 1–48.

Waddington, J. L., Molloy, A. G., O'Boyle, K. M., & Pugh, M. T. (1990). Aspects of stereotyped and non-stereotyped behaviour in relation to dopamine receptor sub-types. In S. J. Cooper & C. T. Dourish (Eds.), *Neurobiology of stereotyped behaviour* (pp. 64–90). Oxford, England: Oxford University Press.

Dopaminergic and Serotonergic Effects on Spontaneous Orofacial Dyskinesias in Cebus Monkeys

Daniel E. Casey

Neuroleptics were first used to treat psychoses in the 1950s. The term *neuroleptic* was developed because of its meaning, "to take the neuron," which implies that the drug took control of neuronal function. Incorporated in the term was the concept that the neuroleptic drugs produced both antipsychotic and motor side effects at the same dose (Delay, Deniker, & Hare, 1952; Deniker, 1984). Therefore, clinicians could identify the appropriate antipsychotic dose by the onset of extrapyramidal symptoms. In the 1960s, this theory was shown to be incorrect; it is well recognized that the neuroleptic drugs have a very narrow therapeutic index. Thus, the majority (approximately 75%) of patients receiving neuroleptic drugs develop signs of motor dysfunction (Casey, 1991b). These include the acute onset disorders of drug-induced dystonia (briefly sustained muscle contractions that lead to abnormal postures), parkinsonism (tremor, rigidity, bradykinesia), and akathisia (subjective or objective signs of restlessness or both), as well as the late onset disorder of tardive dyskinesia (hyperkinetic choreiform dyskinesias; Casey, 1987, 1991b).

Though the neuroleptic drugs are the mainstay of antipsychotic therapy, they are used for other unlabeled indications. Commonly, these drugs are prescribed for persons with stereotypic behavior or severe behavioral disturbances that occur either alone or in the presence of psychoses. However, the efficacy of neuroleptics in these clinical settings is fraught with conflicting data and is a highly controversial subject (Aman, White, & Field, 1984; Heistad, Zimmermann, & Doebler, 1982; Hill, Balow, & Bruininks, 1985; Intagliata & Rinck, 1985; Lewis et al., 1986).

It is curious to note that in addition to reducing stereotyped behavior, neuroleptics can also produce repetitive purposeless behaviors, such as akathisia, a syndrome that is often manifested by stereotyped behavior of shifting from foot to foot, crossing and uncrossing legs, hand wringing, rocking, and so on (Casey, 1991b). Unfortunately, the relationship between neuroleptic-reduced stereotypies and neuroleptic-induced akathisia is not known.

The neuroleptic mechanism of action of the antipsychotic and motor effects is thought to be blockade of the dopamine type 2 (D_2) receptors, which are a subset of the dopamine receptor family classified as D_1, D_2, D_3, D_4, and D_5. This biochemical property is common to all commercially available neuroleptics with antipsychotic and extrapyramidal activity. However, clozapine is a compound that challenges this concept. It has well documented antipsychotic efficacy, but weakly blocks D_1 and D_2 receptors in humans (Farde, Wiesel, Nordström, & Sedvall, 1989). It also produces far fewer acute extrapyramidal symptoms than typical D_2 antagonizing neuroleptics (Casey, 1989a). These data raise important questions about the relative roles of D_1 and D_2 receptors in modulating psychotic symptoms and motor function.

Neuroleptic drugs span several chemical classes and a wide range of low to high milligram potency. In addition, some agents affect multiple neurotransmitters, such as serotonin, acetylcholine, histamine, and noradrenergic systems, producing many undesirable side effects. Ultimately, the goal of new drug development for treating psychoses, stereotypic behavior, and severe behavioral disturbances will be a compound with good clinical efficacy but without any, or far fewer, side effects.

The role of stereotypic behavior in neuroleptic drug development has been crucial. One of the fundamental animal models for screening antipsychotic drugs has been the ability of compounds to block stimulant-induced stereotypic behavior. Hypothetically, this identifies antipsychotic action (Ellinwood, 1971; Ridley, Baker, & Scraggs, 1979). A corresponding model of neuroleptic-induced catalepsy in rodents or dystonia in nonhuman primates identifies the likelihood of a drug producing acute extrapyramidal syndromes (Casey, 1992; Coffin, Latranyi, & Chipkin, 1989). Although these models have been fruitful in identifying many different chemical classes with the dopamine antagonist action in common, they have also been limiting in that drugs with the same type of desirable, as well as undesirable, actions keep being rediscovered by these animal models.

Nonhuman primate models have occasionally been used to evaluate the biochemical basis of stereotypic behavior. Monkeys receiving dopamine-influencing compounds exhibit substantially altered behavior. The most commonly observed behaviors of monkeys receiving dopamine agonists are increasing rates of checking (moving the head from side to side as if checking the environment) and individual repetitive stereotypic behaviors, such as circling, somersaulting, opening and closing the hands, patting the side of the cage repeatedly, and so forth (Casey, Gerlach, & Christensson, 1980b; Lewis, Baumeister, McCorkle, & Mailman, 1985; Ridley et al., 1979; Schlemmer, Narasimhachari, & Davis, 1980).

Nondirect dopamine agonists, such as amphetamine and methylphenidate, have been most commonly studied (Ellinwood, 1971). These drug compounds produce increasing rates of stereotypic behavior with high doses producing an intensely aroused and immobilized animal that may appear to be catatonic because of its apparent immobility. Quite possibly the animal's behavior becomes more narrowly focused as the drug dose rises, so that eventually only one behavior, such as staring from a fixed posture, evolves (Ridley & Baker, 1982). The direct dopamine agonists are somewhat less studied. Selective dopamine D_1 and D_2 agonists have only become available for evaluation in the past few years, though the mixed D_1/D_2 agonist, apomorphine, has been studied for many years. Both receptor subtype agonists produce behavioral syndromes of increased activation, arousal, and stereotypic behavior (Casey & Gerlach, 1986; Casey, Gerlach, & Christensson, 1980a; Gerlach, Casey, & Kistrup, 1986; Gerlach, Casey, Kistrup, & Lublin, 1988; Peacock, Lublin, & Gerlach, 1990).

Similarly, selective D_1 and D_2 antagonists have only recently been developed to provide the opportunity for characterizing the biochemical basis of stereotypies. Antagonists of both receptor subtypes block stereotypic behavior and produce acute extrapyramidal syndromes in monkeys (Casey, 1992; Casey & Gerlach, 1986; Casey et al., 1980b; Coffin et al., 1989; Gerlach et al., 1986; Gerlach et al., 1988; Peacock et al., 1990). With the development of drugs that affect serotonin subtypes of receptors, it is now possible to evaluate the role of serotonin in stereotypic behavior. Drugs that concomitantly block the type-2 receptor subtype of the dopamine (D_2) and serotonin (5-HT2) classes have been proposed as antipsychotic agents with potentially lower extrapyramidal syndrome liability. However, in nonhuman primates these types of drugs have also produced dystonia and parkinsonism (Casey, 1989b, 1991a, 1991c). The critical issue for these new drugs is whether the threshold dose and dose-response curves for antipsychotic and extrapyramidal syndromes are sufficiently separated to provide clinically relevant advantages.

The ability to study new compounds for their potential antistereotypic effects in nondrug-induced stereotypic models has been extremely limited. There are very few animal models that use naturally occurring stereotypic behavior that might be applied to identify potential drugs to treat stereotypies.

The aim of this investigation is to evaluate the role of dopamine and serotonin in spontaneous oral stereotypies in cebus monkeys. The behavior of interest is repetitive tongue protrusions, which occur in the normal behavioral repertoire of some monkeys. These fit the definition of a stereotyped, purposeless, repetitive behavior, and they occur spontaneously so that a nonstimulant-induced behavior could be evaluated.

METHOD

Subjects

Cebus monkeys (14 to 22 years old), with low to moderate rates of spontaneously occurring tongue protrusions that were present before they had received psychotropic compounds, were tested in their home cages.

The time of onset of these behaviors in the monkeys' lives is unknown, however. These stereotypic tongue protrusions were stable in rate (1-3 per 30 s) and intensity. All of the animals received neuroleptic treatment in the several months before the start of this study to establish stable and highly reproducible rates of extrapyramidal syndromes (dystonia and parkinsonism). This required the administration of between 6 and 15 neuroleptic doses spaced several days apart. Without these stable dystonia scores, the study would have suffered from a shifting baseline as the animals eventually achieved their stable responses. Thus, the monkeys met the criteria for being sensitized to neuroleptics. This prior exposure to neuroleptics did not change the baseline rates of tongue protrusions for the monkeys. Also, the stable scores with saline and active drugs in this study indicated that the drug exposures did not alter baseline tongue protrusion rates. The same animals participated in each of the treatment trials.

Drugs

Dopamine and serotonin agonists and antagonists were used to characterize the drug effects on the behaviors of interest. Drugs tested were the D_1 direct, partial agonist SKF38393 (0.5–10 mg/kg); the mixed direct D_1/D_2 agonists apomorphine (0.01–0.25 mg/kg), bromocriptine (0.1–2.5 mg/kg), and pergolide (0.01–0.25 mg/kg); and the indirect agonist amphetamine (0.1–2.5 mg/kg). The specific D_1 antagonist used was SCH23390 (0.01–0.25 mg/kg), and the D_2 antagonists were the butyrophenone haloperidol (0.01–0.25 mg/kg), the substituted benzamide remoxipride (2.5–50 mg/kg), the phenothiazine thioridazine (0.5–10 mg/kg), and risperidone (0.01–0.25 mg/kg). The serotonin 5HT1a agonist was 8-OH DPAT (.025–0.5 mg/kg), and the serotonin 5-HT2 antagonist was ritanserine (0.1–5 mg/kg). Saline control was 0.25 ml volume.

Design

Drugs were tested across a wide dose range and with a saline control. These active and control compounds were given intramuscularly in randomly sequenced doses at 7-day intervals. Each drug and a saline control was fully tested before the next drug was evaluated. It took 6 to 8 weeks to test each drug. There was a 2-week drug-free period between each drug study.

Scoring

Behaviors were scored before and at 15- to 60-min intervals for 6 hr after drug administration by an experienced rater who was blind to drug dose. The behaviors of interest were dystonia and the oral stereotypy of tongue protrusion. Dystonia was scored in four different body areas (head and neck, upper limbs, lower limbs, tail) on a 4-point scale (0 = *none*, 1 = *mild*, 2 = *moderate*, 3 = *severe*). Oral stereotypy was quantified by counting tongue protrusions on three consecutive 30-s periods. Group mean total scores for each behavior are presented in the figures.

RESULTS

Both the specific and nonspecific direct D_1 and D_2 agonists had only a modest effect on tongue protrusion. SKF38393, apomorphine, bromocriptine, and pergolide did not appreciably change tongue protrusion rates from the spontaneously occurring level rated during the saline control test. However, the nondirect, nonspecific agonist, amphetamine, dose-relatedly decreased the spontaneous tongue protrusions down to complete suppression at 0.5, 1, and 2.5 mg/kg. None of the D_1 and D_2 agonists produced dystonia (see Figure 1).

The D_1 antagonist, SCH23390, did not appreciably affect the oral stereotypy of tongue protrusion, though there was a modest trend to a decrease from saline control levels with increasing drug doses. However, SCH23390 did produce a dose-related dystonia syndrome. Haloperidol, remoxipride, and risperidone all produced dose-related decreases in the oral stereotypy, but only at the doses that also produced dose-related onset and increased dystonic syndromes. Thioridazine reduced tongue protrusions at the cost of dystonia, but the dystonic syndromes were less severe than those with the other D_2 antagonists (see Figure 2).

The serotonin 1-A agonist, 8-OH DPAT, dose-relatedly suppressed oral stereotypies down to 0 at 0.5 mg/kg, and no dystonia was produced. Similarly, the serotonin 5-HT2 antagonist, ritanserine, dose-relatedly de-

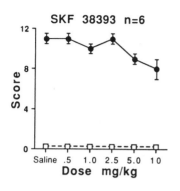

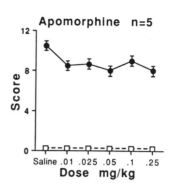

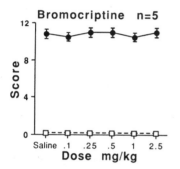

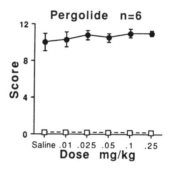

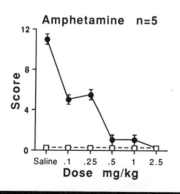

Figure 1

The effect of dopamine D_1 (SKF38393) and D_2 agonists on spontaneous tongue protrusions and dystonia. ● = tongue protrusions and □ = dystonia.

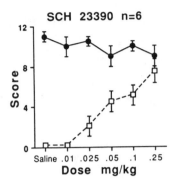

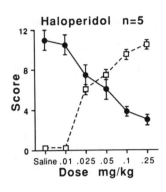

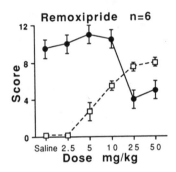

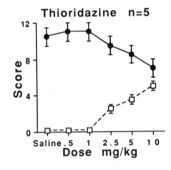

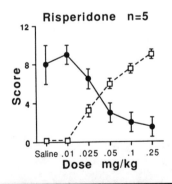

Figure 2

The effect of dopamine D_1 (SCH23390) and D_2 antagonists on spontaneous tongue protrusions and dystonia. ● = tongue protrusions and □ = dystonia.

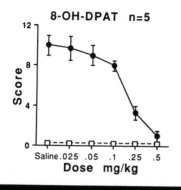
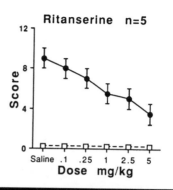

Figure 3

The effect of a serotonin 5-HT1a agonist (8-OH DPAT) and 5-HT2 antagonist (ritanserine) on spontaneous tongue protrusions and dystonia.

creased stereotypic tongue protrusions down to 50% of saline control levels. Neither compound produced dystonia (see Figure 3).

CONCLUSION

The stereotypic behavior of spontaneously occurring, repetitive tongue protrusions in nonhuman primates may be a useful model of human stereotypies. It has the advantage of being a stereotyped behavior that occurs spontaneously and does not require stimulant induction, as do many other nonhuman primate stereotyped behaviors. Though these repetitive behaviors, which occur in a distinct minority (5%-10%) of cebus monkeys, appear to be purposeless, it is not possible to know if there is a goal-directed intent to the tongue protrusion activity. Other species also develop stereotyped behavior in the natural setting, such as licking syndromes in cows and dogs. These may provide additional models for studying the much underinvestigated nature of stereotyped activities.

Dopamine has a complex role in modulating oral stereotypic tongue protrusion. The D_1 and D_2 specific or mixed agonists had no strikingly consistent effect on tongue protrusions, with the exception of amphetamine, which dose-relatedly decreased this behavior. This decrease may identify some action unique to amphetamine, or it may merely be that amphetamine produced such an increased rate of arousal and limited repertoire of behavior that tongue protrusions dropped out of the normal complex behavior group as other, more limited behaviors predominated. However, the high doses of amphetamine required to produce these effects preclude its usefulness in the clinical setting. Neither dopamine D_1 agonism nor antagonism had much effect on oral stereotypies. This suggests that the D_1 dopamine system does not have a primary role in regulating this oral stereotypic behavior and, by implication, indicates that drugs acting via D_1 mechanisms may not be effective in reducing stereotypic behaviors seen in the clinic. This conclusion must remain tentative until other compounds in this class are studied and generalizations about multiple agents with D_1 actions can be made.

Though it initially appears that the lack of dopamine agonist effects conflicts with earlier reports, this may not be the case. In most other studies, the effect of agonists in provoking stereotypic behavior was evaluated, whereas the present investigation evaluated spontaneously occurring oral stereotypies. The prior observations of dopamine agonist–induced competing behaviors may explain why some existing behaviors remain unchanged or actually decrease, as was seen with amphetamine in this study, while new drug-related activities are provoked. In the clinical setting, there are very few data about the acute effects of dopamine agonists on baseline stereotypic behavior with which to compare the results of this investigation. In chronic amphetamine or other stimulant use in humans and monkeys, there is a decrease in normal behaviors while remaining behaviors become increasingly stereotyped (Ellinwood, 1971).

The traditional dopamine D_2 antagonists all suppressed the oral stereotypy, but at the trade-off cost of causing drug-induced dystonia. This observation parallels clinical findings, in which the neuroleptic drugs from several different chemical classes are used to treat psychosis or stereotypic behavior, but are often limited by their drug-induced motor syndromes (Casey, 1991b). Interestingly, thioridazine, a neuroleptic that is commonly used to treat stereotyped behavior in individuals with developmental disabilities (Heistad et al., 1982), appears to have the ability to partially reduce oral stereotypies without producing incapacitating levels of dystonia or other extrapyramidal syndromes in nonhuman primates. However, this effect occurs within only a very narrow dose range, suggesting that many patients with stereotypic behavior will have extrapyramidal symptoms when treated with standard thioridazine doses.

Data from the present study also suggest that serotonin may have an important role in the cause and potential treatment of human stereotypies. Serotonin 5HT1a activation with the agonist 8-OH DPAT produced complete suppression of oral stereotypic tongue protrusion. Ritanserine, a serotonin 5-HT2 antagonist, appeared to have only partial efficacy in suppressing oral dyskinesias, though higher doses might produce a greater response. In both these drug classes, there was no dystonia produced by either compound. These data suggest that perhaps stereotypies occur from imbalances in the serotonin regulatory processes. If so, reestablishing proper serotonin tone with serotonergic agents may be a mechanism for treating stereotypic behavior. Support for this proposal comes from the findings that the selective serotonin reuptake inhibitors are helpful in treating obsessive–compulsive disorders. Further pursuing the development and testing of compounds with these types of serotonergic actions in clinical populations with stereotypic behavior may be a fruitful line of investigation that will lead to greater clinical efficacy with fewer side effects.

REFERENCES

Aman, M. G., White, A. J., & Field, C. (1984). Chlorpromazine effects on stereotypic and conditioned behavior of severely retarded patients—A pilot study. *Journal of Mental Deficiency Research, 28,* 253–260.

Casey, D. E. (1987). Tardive dyskinesia. In H. Meltzer (Ed.), *Psychopharmacology: The third generation of progress* (pp. 1411–1419). New York: Raven.

Casey, D. E. (1989a). Clozapine: Neuroleptic-induced EPS and tardive dyskinesia. *Psychopharmacology, 99,* S47–S53.

Casey, D. E. (1989b). Serotonergic aspects of acute extrapyramidal syndromes in nonhuman primates. *Psychopharmacology Bulletin, 25,* 457–459.

Casey, D. E. (1991a). Extrapyramidal syndromes in nonhuman primates: Typical and atypical neuroleptics. *Psychopharmacology Bulletin, 27,* 47–50.

Casey, D. E. (1991b). Neuroleptic drug-induced extrapyramidal syndromes and tardive dyskinesia. *Schizophrenia Research, 4,* 109–120.

Casey, D. E. (1991c). Serotonin and dopamine relationships in nonhuman primate extrapyramidal syndromes. *Journal of the European College of Neuropsychopharmacology, S15-3*, 351–353.

Casey, D. E. (1992). Dopamine D_1 (SCH23390) and D_2 (haloperidol) antagonists in drug-naive monkeys. *Psychopharmacology, 107*, 18–22.

Casey, D. E., & Gerlach, J. (1986). Is tardive dyskinesia due to dopamine hypersensitivity? *Clinical Neuropharmacology, 9* (Suppl. 4), 134–136.

Casey, D. E., Gerlach, J., & Christensson, E. (1980a). Behavioral aspects of GABA–dopamine interrelationships in the monkey. *Brain Research Bulletin, 5* (Suppl. 2), 269–273.

Casey, D. E., Gerlach, J., & Christensson, E. (1980b). Dopamine, acetylcholine, and GABA effects in acute dystonia in primates. *Psychopharmacology, 70*, 83–87.

Coffin, V. L., Latranyi, M. B., & Chipkin, R. E. (1989). Acute extrapyramidal syndrome in cebus monkeys: Development mediated by dopamine D_2 but not D_1 receptors. *Journal of Pharmacology and Experimental Therapeutics, 249*, 769–774.

Delay, J., Deniker, P., & Hare, J. M. (1952). Utilisation en therapeutique psychiatrique d'une phenothiazine d'action centrale elective (4560 RP). [The psychiatric therapeutic effect of a centrally acting phenothiazine (4560 RP)]. *Annales Medicopsychologiques, 110*, 112–117.

Deniker, P. (1984). Introduction of neuroleptic chemotherapy into psychiatry. In F. J. Ayd & B. Blackwell (Eds.), *Discoveries in biological psychiatry* (pp. 155–164). Baltimore: Ayd Medical Communications.

Ellinwood, E. H. (1971). Effect of chronic methamphetamine intoxication in rhesus monkeys. *Biological Psychiatry, 3*, 25–32.

Farde, L., Wiesel, F. A., Nordström, A. L., & Sedvall, G. (1989). D_1- and D_2-dopamine receptor occupancy during treatment with conventional and atypical neuroleptics. *Psychopharmacology, 99*, S28–S31.

Gerlach, J., Casey, D. E., & Kistrup, K. (1986). D_1 and D_2 receptor manipulation in cebus monkeys: Implication for extrapyramidal syndromes in humans. *Clinical Neuropharmacology, 9* (Suppl. 4), 131–133.

Gerlach, J., Casey, D. E., Kistrup, K., & Lublin, H. (1988). Dopamine D_1 and D_2 receptor functions in acute extrapyramidal syndromes and tardive dyskinesia. In R. H. Belmaker, M. Sandler, & A. Dahlstrom (Eds.), *Neurology and neurobiology* (Vol. 42C, pp. 1–4). New York: Alan R. Liss.

Heistad, G. T., Zimmermann, R. L., & Doebler, M. I. (1982). Long-term usefulness of thioridazine for institutionalized mentally retarded patients. *American Journal of Mental Deficiency, 87*, 243–251.

Hill, B. K., Balow, E. A., & Bruininks, R. H. (1985). A national study of prescribed drugs in institutions and community residential facilities for mentally retarded people. *Psychopharmacology Bulletin, 21,* 279–284.

Intagliata, J., & Rinck, C. (1985). Psychoactive drug use in public and community residential facilities for mentally retarded persons. *Psychopharmacology Bulletin, 21,* 268–278.

Lewis, M. H., Baumeister, A. A., McCorkle, D.L., & Mailman, R. B. (1985). A computer supported method for analyzing behavioral observations: Studies with stereotypy. *Psychopharmacology, 85,* 204–209.

Lewis, M. H., Steer, R. A., Favell, J., McGimsey, J., Clontz, L., Trivette, C., Jodry, W., Schroeder, S., Kanoy, R., & Mailman, R. B. (1986). Thioridazine metabolism and effects on stereotyped behavior in mentally retarded patients. *Psychopharmacology Bulletin, 22,* 1040–1044.

Peacock, L., Lublin, H., & Gerlach, J. (1990). The effects of dopamine D_1 and D_2 receptor agonists and antagonists in monkeys withdrawn from long-term neuroleptic treatment. *European Journal of Pharmacology, 186,* 49–59.

Ridley, R. M., & Baker, H. F. (1982). Stereotypy in monkeys and humans. *Psychological Medicine, 12,* 61–72.

Ridley, R. F., Baker, H. F., & Scraggs, P. R. (1979). The time course of the behavioral effects of amphetamine and their reversal by haloperidol in a primate species. *Biological Psychiatry, 14,* 753–765.

Schlemmer, R. F., Jr., Narasimhachari, N., & Davis, J. M. (1980). Dose-dependent behavioural changes induced by apomorphine in selected members of a primate social colony. *Journal of Pharmacy and Pharmacology, 32,* 285–289.

PART THREE

Measuring the
Movements

5

Instruments for Assessing Stereotypic Movements: A Review of the Literature

Robert L. Sprague

A quote from a well-known researcher provides a good introduction to this chapter. Child psychiatrist Magda Campbell is distinguished for her years of research on autism and more recent research on differentially diagnosing abnormal movements, stereotypies, and tardive dyskinesia in children. A few years ago, she and a colleague wrote, "Appropriate assessment instruments should be selected on the basis of their known validity, reliability, and sensitivity to drug effects" (Campbell & Deutsch, 1985, p. 216). The concepts they enunciated are as sound now as they were at the time of writing. This appropriate emphasis on psychometric properties, often missing in clinical research, was one of the reasons this chapter was prepared. In the absence of empirical data on psychometric properties, the clinical data on prevalence, severity, and so on, are often of limited value because each clinician tends to have her or his own internal standard. Thus, the author undertook a review of assessment procedures for tardive dyskinesia.

SYMPTOMS OF TARDIVE DYSKINESIA

As defined in the introduction to this book, *stereotyped movements* are repeated movement sequences that appear to the observer to have no obvious goal. There are a number of disorders producing stereotyped movements, but this chapter will be limited to examining movements primarily
caused by environmental deprivation resulting in a display of stereotyped
movements and *tardive dyskinesia* (TD). TD is an abnormal involuntary
movement disorder caused by long-term use of psychoactive medications,
usually neuroleptic drugs.

TD has been described in many articles, perhaps the best of which is
contained in a book published by a psychiatric organization (American
Psychiatric Association [APA], 1979). Before the complete syndrome of
TD develops, there are early indicators: fine movements of the tongue in
the mouth; frequent bursts of blinking, tic-like movements of the lips or
face; and slight involuntary jerky movements of the fingers and/or hands.
If the disorder progresses, other facial movements often begin; these include protrusion of the tongue outside the mouth, sucking or smacking
lip movements, arching of the eyebrows, grimacing of the face. Other parts
of the body often display abnormal involuntary movements such as rest-
less, jerky, or slowly twisting movements of the hand, fingers, and sometimes toes; tapping of the feet; backward jerking of the head for several
seconds to minutes; turning of the head to one side; and rocking, swaying, and shoulder shrugging in the trunk of the body.

At present, there is no consensus for an effective treatment of TD
(APA, 1979). Often the disorder remains with the patient for many years,
sometimes for life. Considering the lack of an effective treatment and the
long-term nature of the disorder, it is important to diagnose the disorder
early and take action to prevent the development of the full-blown syndrome. Thus, there is considerable emphasis in the medical literature on
prevention of TD, which takes several forms. Primary prevention involves
using neuroleptic drugs only for appropriate clinical conditions and then
using them in the lowest doses that are clinically effective. Secondary prevention is considered to involve using periodic, systematic examinations

to detect the earliest symptoms of the development of TD. Therefore, reliable, valid, and sensitive measures of the earliest symptoms of TD are quite valuable to the prevention of the disorder. Because there is no laboratory test for TD, the emphasis is placed on observational measures to detect the earliest symptoms. Psychometric properties of these observational behavioral measures, thus, become important factors in the prevention of the disorder. The remainder of this chapter is devoted to consideration of the psychometric properties of measures of abnormal movement disorders.

STANDARDS FOR BEHAVIORAL ASSESSMENTS

Surprisingly little attention has been paid to the details of adequate standards for assessment instruments in this important area of monitoring abnormal movements of patient populations. Although lip-service is sometimes paid to psychometrics of instrument development, the training of users, and use with specified populations, instruments for measuring tardive dyskinetic movements have generally not been scrutinized from the viewpoint of psychometric standards. These difficulties have been recognized since 1977. At that time Gardos, Cole, and La Brie (1977) published an insightful review of the assessment of TD. They prophetically wrote,

> [U]ntil a breakthrough in the therapy of dyskinesia is achieved, the refining of current assessment methods and the selection of appropriate measuring tools for a given research study would go a long way toward increasing knowledge about this heterogeneous and puzzling condition. (p. 1212)

Two of these authors writing 3 years later (Gardos & Cole, 1980) cogently pointed out, "[T]here should be specific operational criteria for defining tardive dyskinesia" (p. 206). The hoped-for "breakthrough" has not been found (APA, 1992), and there has not been much "refining" of TD assessment techniques.

Several years ago, three professional organizations joined forces to develop and issue *Standards for Educational and Psychological Testing* (American Educational Research Association [AERA], 1985).[1] Because there has been little discussion of psychometric standards in the TD literature, it will be helpful to list and examine 21 of the principles from *Standards* that my colleagues and I believe are appropriate to assess abnormal movements (Sprague, 1985, 1986, 1988):

1.1 "Evidence of validity should be presented" (p. 13).

1.2 "If validity for some common interpretations has not been investigated, that fact should be made clear" (p. 13).

1.4 "Whenever it is suggested that the user consider an individual's responses to specific items as a basis for assessment, the test manual should present . . . evidence" (p. 14).

1.5 "The composition of the validation sample should be described" (p. 14).

1.7 "When . . . experts have been asked to judge . . . the items . . . , the relevant training, experience, and qualifications of the experts should be described" (p. 15).

1.8 "When a test is proposed as a measure of a construct, that construct should be distinguished from other constructs" (p. 15).

1.11 "A report of a criterion-related validation study should provide a description of the sample and the statistical analysis used" (p. 16).

1.24 "If specific cut scores are recommended for decision making, . . . the user's guide should caution that the rates of misclassification will vary depending on the percentage of individuals tested . . . in each category" (p. 18).

2.1 "For each total score, subscore, or combination of scores that is reported, estimates of relevant reliabilities and standard errors of measurement should be provided" (p. 20).

---

[1]These organizations, which have a professional interest in maintaining the highest standards for tests, are the American Educational Research Association, the American Psychological Association, and the National Council on Measurement in Education. The book was published by the American Psychological Association and contains 100 pages of detailed standards and procedures for every phase of test construction, development, training of users, and use with specified populations. A total of 180 standards are listed in this book, which is more detail than would be useful here. Excerpts from *Standards for Educational and Psychological Testing.* Copyright 1985 by the American Psychological Association. Reprinted with permission of the publisher.

2.2   "The procedures that are used to obtain samples . . . should be described" (p. 20).

2.8   "When judgmental processes enter into the scoring . . . evidence on the degree of agreement . . . should be provided" (p. 22).

3.1   "Tests and testing programs should be developed on a sound scientific basis" (p. 20).

3.4   "When test items relate to a course of training . . . , the manual . . . should include . . . [a] description of the course" (p. 26).

3.18   "A test should be . . . revised" (p. 29).

3.21   "The directions for test administration should be presented" (p. 29).

4.1   "Scales used . . . and the rationale for choosing them should be described" (p. 33).

4.4   "Reports of norming studies should include the year in which normative data were collected" (p. 33).

5.2   "Test manuals should describe thoroughly the rationale for the test, . . . and provide a summary of the support for such uses" (p. 36).

5.4   "Test manuals should identify any special qualifications that are required to administer a test" (p. 36).

6.9   "When a specific cut score is used . . . , the method . . . for setting that cut score should be presented" (p. 43).

7.3   "When differential diagnosis is needed, . . . evidence of the test's ability to distinguish between . . . diagnostic groups [should be reported]" (p. 46).

Although no research group that has worked with rating scales for TD, including our own group, has met all of these high standards, the standards do provide a goal toward which researchers should strive. Without attention to such psychometric goals, it is not likely that the level of assessment in the TD field will quickly advance. The literature contains widely discrepant estimates of the prevalence of TD in populations of patients exposed to neuroleptic medications. This important question of prevalence and other equally pressing issues can best be answered with psychometrically sound instruments.

REVIEW OF LITERATURE FROM
A PSYCHOMETRIC PERSPECTIVE

In a quote that is, if anything, an understatement of the literature regarding TD assessment techniques, Simpson and Singh (1988) stated, "There are methodological problems with most of the studies which address the epidemiology of TD. The problems include lack of an acceptable and clinically useful criteria for the diagnosis of TD [sic]. . . . The problems with the global items used in rating scales [are] that their validity, reliability and sensitivity are apt to be poor" (p. 176). In a discussion of training of raters, the authors stated, "Another problem . . . is that . . . specific instructions for rating procedures are lacking" (p. 176). Finally, in relation to the stability of TD scores over time, the authors cogently pointed out the need for such information: "A critically troublesome problem in the assessment of TD is the tendency for its manifestations to undergo extensive fluctuations. . . . [T]here are . . . patients who show marked fluctuation in movements from day to day" (p. 179). In this important article regarding TD rating scales, Simpson and Singh pointed out numerous general problems in the assessment of TD using rating scale instruments; however, they often failed to give specific details about psychometric data for the rating scales they mentioned. In addition, there are some rating scales with psychometric data that the authors did not mention. This chapter is an attempt to provide some of the information not contained in their article.

It has been difficult to locate studies that evaluate the psychometric aspects of TD rating scales. Much of the literature has addressed the pressing clinical questions of screening for TD, influence of various medications on the TD symptoms, possible risk factors involved with the development of TD, and similar clinical issues. One good example of this orientation to the assessment of TD is one of the comprehensive reviews of the literature written by Jeste and Wyatt (1982). Although the book is long and has numerous chapters covering a variety of topics, it has very limited information on the psychometrics of the rating scales reviewed. For example, the following relevant topics cannot be found in the otherwise helpful index: measurement, rating scale, reliability, interrater reliability, psychometrics, sensitivity, stability, or validity.[2]

It is now commonly accepted in science and medicine that a basic aspect of understanding a disease is measurement of the symptoms or, at least, emphasis on measurement of the symptoms in order to improve diagnostic accuracy. Lack of such an emphasis in the TD literature is perplexing.

In the most recent and probably best book on the topic (APA, 1992), a similar gap can be seen. There are some improvements from the perspective of psychometric issues. However, the index also lacks the terms previously cited for the Jeste and Wyatt (1982) book, although reliability and validity issues are covered. There are also sections on rating methods and multi-item scales and a table listing 14 rating scales, but there are no comparative psychometric data given for the scales.

In addition to this lack of interest in the psychometric properties of the instruments used to measure the number and severity of TD symptoms, it is also quite difficult to find literature presenting data on reliability and validity because the psychometrically relevant topical words previously listed are generally not used in the abstracts of articles dealing with TD. This means such terms are typically not included in the various reference databases available. For the present project, it was necessary to search the general literature on TD with the hope of finding articles that address some of these psychometric issues. Thus, this review is not exhaustive because articles might have been missed because of the problems noted above. Table 1 presents an overall summary of the studies reviewed.

AIMS

The Abnormal Involuntary Movement Scale (AIMS) has been widely accepted probably because it was the first instrument in the area and because it was published in a National Institute of Mental Health publication (Guy, 1976).

---

[2]These topics are missing in the index even though the two most widely used rating scales (Abnormal Involuntary Movement Scale and Rockland Research Institute [Simpson] Abbreviated Dyskinesia Rating Scale) are discussed at some length.

Table 1

Psychometric Properties of Instruments

Study	Number of Subjects	Number of Raters	Interrater Reliability	Validity	Rater Training
Abnormal Involuntary Movement Scale					
Ahrens et al., 1988	390	13	correlation .96	—	—
Bergen et al., 1984	4	3	6 correlations .90 to .97	—	—
Germer et al., 1984	2	4	correlation .97	—	videotape
Guy, Ban, & Wilson, 1985	768	—	—	clinical & RD/TD correlation .39	—
Lane et al., 1985	33		9 correlations .46 to .81	—	—
Richardson & Craig, 1982	132	1	—	16 AIMS & Simpson correlations 15 significant, total score .98	—
Smith et al., 1979	213	3	9 correlations .35 to .89	—	videotape
Smith et al., 1979	39–48	4	9 correlations .66 to .87	—	videotape
Barnes Scale					
Barnes, Rossor, & Thauer, 1983	310	3	8 stability correlations .92 to .99	patients had significantly higher scores on ratings	—
Barnes & Trauer, 1982	94	3	8 correlations .83 to .99	correlation with AIMS .63	videotape

Berkson and Davenport Stereotypy Checklist

Berkson, 1964	50	—	agreement 29% to 96%	—	—
	48	—			—
Berkson, 1965	4	—	—	medication had no significant effect	—
Berkson & Davenport, 1962	71	2	correlations .76 to .95 stability correlations .26 to .53	age correlates .33, IQ − .31	—
Berkson & Mason, 1963	14	2	4 correlations .74 to .99	situations significantly different	—
Berkson & Mason, 1964	15	—	—	situations significantly different	—
	25	—	—	correlation − .40 with object manipulation	—
	27	—	3 correlations .79 to .85	—	—
	35	—	—	ratings significantly interacted with environment	—
Davenport & Berkson, 1963	24	—	—	situations significantly different	—

DISCUS

Kalachnik, Harder, et al., 1984	191	14	—	medication withdrawal significantly increased ratings	—

(table continues)

Table 1 (*Continued*)

Psychometric Properties of Instruments

Study	Number of Subjects	Number of Raters	Interrater Reliability	Validity	Rater Training
			DISCUS		
Kalachnik, Sprague, & Slaw, 1988	263	—	—	significant effect of training	14 workshops and video-tapes
Sprague, Kalachnik, et al., 1984	177	14	34 correlations .14 to .81, total .78; 34 stability correlations −.03 to .65, total .77	—	—
Sprague et al., 1989	148	2	16 correlations .42 to .79, total .92; 16 stability correlations .10 to .75	—	12-hr class videotape
Sprague & Kalachnik, 1991	277	92	16 correlations .45 to .91, total .92	diagnosed cases were significantly higher than nondiagnosed	workshops and video-tapes
	407	128	16 correlations .57 to .97, total .91		
Sprague et al., 1993	36	—	—	pattern of correlations with dynamic measures	—

Sct. Hans Scale

Study	N		Reliability	Validity	
Hoffman et al., 1987	21	—	—	no significant multiple correlation	—

Simpson Tardive Dyskinesia Rating Scale

Study	N		Reliability	Validity	
Albus et al., 1985	36	2	—	CT scans correlate .54	—
Firth & Arden, 1985	10	2	agreement 75% to 91%	—	—
Izumi et al., 1986	11	—	—	meclofenoxate reduced ratings	—
Richardson & Craig, 1982	132	1	—	16 AIMS & Simpson correlations	—
Simpson et al. 1979	26	2	correlations .55 to .99	15 significant, total score .98	—
	23	9	interrater correlation .79 to .99		—
			videotape correlation .87 to .91		—

Note: — indicates information not provided in study.

In a study of 390 patients, Ahrens, Sramek, Herrera, Jewett, and Alcorn (1988) obtained a summary interrater reliability correlation on the AIMS of .96 "between the primary rater and 12 staff physicians" (p. 206) for 60 randomly selected patients. Because there are no details given as to how this summary correlation was obtained, questions arise owing to the fact that correlation coefficients should not be added together and then divided by the number of pairs of ratings to obtain an average correlation. The correlations should be transformed using the Fisher's z and then averaged (Cohen & Cohen, 1975). Several of the studies reviewed in this chapter do not report whether the proper transformation was done before the average correlation was calculated, which places the reliability data from these studies in question.

Bergen, Griffiths, Rey, and Beumont (1984) studied only 4 outpatients over a period of time that was not specified. The estimated duration of neuroleptic treatment ranged from 17 to 22 years. Three psychiatrists "experienced in assessment of TD" (p. 498) rated three of the subjects 11 different times and one subject 13 times. From this matrix of raters at different examination times, 48 correlations were obtained. The correlations varied from a high of .97 on AIMS item 4 for two of the raters, to a low of .48 on item 7 for another two raters. The total score yielded higher interrater reliability correlations than individual items. The total score reliability between pairs of raters varied from a low of .90 to a high of .97. The stability of one rater over 6 weeks was reported as a range of .63 to .95; the total score was .94.

Germer, Seraydarian, and McBrearty (1984) trained 15 psychiatrists, 15 nurses, and 9 physicians in a 3-hour videotape training session. Few details are given on how these 39 people rated the videotapes of only two patients. The reported interrater reliability alpha coefficient was .97.

A study of schizophrenic patients from Hungary was conducted by Gardos, Perenyi, Cole, Samu, and Kallos (1983). In 1978, 122 patients were evaluated by one of the authors using the AIMS and Simpson instruments, and 3 years later 47 of the patients were examined again. The authors stated, "No significant changes occurred during the 3 years" (p. 315). From one perspective, this study provides some stability data on these two instruments. On the AIMS all the scores increased; the total score increased 1.34 points.

In what is clearly the largest study of a validity indicator for the AIMS, Guy, Ban, and Wilson (1985) included 768 chronic schizophrenic patients from 11 different mental health centers in eight countries. Few details are presented on how the ratings of the patients were made, who made the ratings, or what the training and experience of the raters were. The AIMS was scored for TD according to the RD/TD of Schooler and Kane (1982), which requires a severity score of 2 on at least one item of the AIMS, or a score of 1 on two different items. Clinical diagnoses of TD were made by psychiatrists at each of the centers. The evidence for validity of the AIMS as indicated by its correlation with the clinical diagnosis was quite low at .39. There are a number of problems interpreting this experiment. It is not known whether the low correlation was due to the possibly limited experience or lack of training of the raters, the probably low reliability of the clinical diagnosis, the lack of validity of the AIMS, some combination of these factors, or possibly other variables. Nevertheless, in this study of the AIMS with the largest sample of subjects, the evidence for the validity of the AIMS rating scale is meager indeed.

In a study of 33 outpatients, Lane, Glazer, Hansen, Berman, and Kramer (1985) randomly selected a patient to rate each week for about 10 months. Four psychiatrists participated as the raters, at least three of whom independently rated the outpatient in each weekly session except for one session. Although it was not explained exactly how the correlations were obtained on the entire group of outpatients, 9 correlations are reported: seven for the body areas, one for the severity rating, and one for the total scores. The lowest correlation is .60 for the lips, and the highest is .81 for the total score. Because the raters were two experienced psychiatrists very familiar with the AIMS and TD and two residents with "minimal prior exposure to . . . TD" (p. 354), it is surprising that the correlations were not higher than those obtained. In comparison with most of the other studies, the experience of the researchers combined with training of the residents should have produced the highest reliability correlations that one could reasonably expect.

Richardson and Craig (1982) modified slightly the AIMS and the Simpson Tardive Dyskinesia Rating Scale so that the two scales could be directly compared in a validity study they conducted. Only one rater examined 132 patients with both scales, which makes the generalizability from this study problematical. Because several raters typically examine patients over time, it is essential that some data be obtained on more than one rater if the reader is interested in the validity of the scale in a clinical situation. Scores for three body areas and a total score were obtained for each scale, which generated 16 correlations. The lowest was total trunk of the Simpson Scale with total extremities of the AIMS at .10; the highest was total facial of both scales of .98.

There are few studies using the AIMS with mentally retarded people. One of the best studies was written by Richardson, Haugland, Pass, and Craig (1986). From the resident population of an institution, 211 people were examined by two raters using the AIMS. Reliability data were obtained for two raters on a sample of 25 residents; the correlations varied from a low of .79 to a high of .93. As is commonly known, there is considerable overlap between the symptoms of TD caused by neuroleptic medication and stereotyped movements believed to be caused by social deprivation and other environmental factors. This study indicated that overlap: the RD/TD criteria (discussed previously in the Guy et al. [1985] review) were significantly related to stereotypic rocking ($X^2 = 23.00$; $p < .001$). A significant canonical correlation of .53 was found between TD and the variables of age, disorders of metabolism, psychosocial deprivation, and gender.

In the best designed study of the reliability of the AIMS, Smith, Kucharski, Oswald, and Waterman (1979) examined 377 patients using four raters. Every patient was rated independently by at least two raters. The raters were trained using a videotape and practiced on 9 patients before beginning the experiment. Interrater reliability was assessed in a group of 39 to 48 patients who were rated twice, 7 weeks apart. The average correlation on the team ratings was calculated using Fisher's z transformation for the seven body areas plus severity and total score. The highest reliability correlation was .87 for the total score and the lowest was .66 for the facial item.

A study of interrater reliability was conducted by Smith, Kucharski, Eblen, Knutsen, and Linn (1979) in a population of 213 patients. The three raters were trained using a videotape. The raters worked in pairs to rate independently all of the participating patients; one pair rated 80 patients, another pair rated 64, and the third pair rated 69. Average correlations were obtained for the teams using Fisher's z transformation. The lowest reliability correlation was .35 over 80 patients for the facial item, and the highest correlation was .89 for 64 patients on the total score. Combining all the ratings, again the lowest correlation was for the facial item at .48 and the highest for total score .87.

Barnes Scale

Barnes and Trauer (1982) developed a rating scale for TD using a videotape procedure. The scale contains eight body areas and is rated on a 4-point scale from 0 (*absent*) to 3 (*continuous movement*). A group of three raters viewed videotapes of 94 patients, then viewed the same videotapes 6 weeks later. The stability-over-time correlations for the three raters over the eight body areas varied from a high of .99 for the three items of neck, trunk, and arms to a low of .82 for the lip item. In a test of interrater reliability, these three raters were compared with three new raters using the second set of videotapes for the patients. The eight interrater reliability correlations varied from .83 for the lip item to .99 for the neck. A validity indicator was taken as the modal rating of the three raters cast into four categories of TD (absent, mild, moderate, and severe) obtained from the Barnes Scale in comparison to similar categories obtained by the raters on the AIMS. The phi correlation was .63.

Barnes, Kidger, and Gore (1983) videotaped 120 outpatients who were receiving neuroleptic medication. The videotapes were judged by three independent raters. After a period of 3 years, 99 of the original group were videotaped again. The large set of data was analyzed several different ways using a distribution of the scores by age band as the primary means of analysis. A logistic regression model was used to ascertain relationship between the two sets of ratings. The best predictor of the presence of TD in the second evaluation was evidence of TD in the earlier evaluation conducted 3 years previously, which indicates some stability of the measurement over several years.

Barnes, Rossor, and Trauer (1983) videotaped a group of 310 subjects: 182 psychiatric patients, 85 normal people, and 43 elderly psychiatric patients. Three raters viewed the videotapes. Patients had significantly higher scores than control ($F = 9.7$; $df = 1, 1855$; $p < .0001$), and there was a significant interaction of body sites and groups ($F = 3.56$; $df = 7, 1855$; $p < .005$).

Berkson and Davenport Stereotypy Checklist

In the area of stereotyped behaviors primarily due to social deprivation, only one instrument has received much research attention—the Berkson and Davenport Stereotypy Checklist. Berkson and Davenport (1962) investigated the stereotyped movements of 71 institutionalized mentally retarded people. The initial checklist contained 10 different types of behavior analyzed in three categories of behavior: self-manipulations, manipulation of the environment, and stereotyped movements. The interrater reliability correlations for two raters calculated on two different days varied from a low of .76 for self-manipulation on day 1 and stereotyped behavior on day 2, to a high of .95 for manipulation of the environment on day 2. The stability correlation over 1 week varied from a low of .26 for self-manipulation to a high of .53 for stereotyped behavior. As validity indicators for the checklist, the checklist categories were correlated with age, IQ, and length of institutionalization. The six significant correlations varied from a low of $-.31$ for stereotyped behaviors and IQ to a high of .33 for stereotyped behaviors and the other two variables, age and length of institutionalization.

Davenport and Berkson (1963) studied 24 institutionalized mentally retarded people in several situations using the checklist. A group of high- and low-stereotyped subjects were selected and examined in seven different situations. The high-stereotyped group engaged in significantly more stereotyped behavior in three situations in which there were no objects present. In contrast, the low-stereotyped group engaged in significantly more exploration behavior in four situations in which objects were available. These effects indicated that the checklist was valid for indicating the interaction of the stereotyped behavior and environmental factors.

Berkson and Mason (1963) investigated the effects of three different environments on stereotyped behavior in 14 profoundly retarded male residents using two raters. Interrater reliability correlations varied from .74 to .99. Validity for the checklist was indicated by a significant interaction between categories of stereotyped behavior and the three environments ($F = 2.18$; $df = 42, 42$).

Berkson and Mason (1964) reported four experiments. In the first experiment, 15 institutionalized mentally retarded people were studied in four situations. There was a significant effect ($F = 5.68$; $df = 3, 42$) of situations on rated stereotyped behavior, which indicated the checklist has some validity for examining the social effects of different environments.

In the second experiment, 25 institutionalized residents were studied. The checklist behaviors correlated $-.40$ with manipulation of objects in the environment, which, again, indicates the checklist has some validity.

Reliability of the checklist was addressed again in the third experiment. A total of 27 institutionalized mentally retarded men were included in the experiment. Reliability correlations of three measures over two sessions were reported: number of intervals in which objects were manipulated (.79), number of objects manipulated (.85), and sum of number of intervals (.77).

In the fourth experiment, 35 residents were divided into three groups: no stereotyped movements, rocking movements, and complex movements. The environmental manipulations significantly changed ratings of self-manipulation ($p = < .005$). More interestingly, the environmental changes significantly interacted with the ratings: for the no-stereotyped-movement group, there was a reduction in locomotion ($p < .05$), and for the complex-movements group, locomotion was increased ($p = < .05$). The rocking-movements group manipulated objects more than the complex movements group ($p = < .05$).

The fourth study in this series (Berkson, 1964) involved a normative experiment with 50 males similar to those subjects described previously. Both interrater reliability and stability over time from 1 day to 7 days were reported. The percentage agreement between two raters varied from a low of 29% for words spoken to a high of 96% for body postures. The stability correlations varied from a low of .26 for number of objects to a high of .96 for words spoken. The authors also published the list of 10 behaviors contained in the checklist and, more important, they provided the definitions of the behaviors. In effect, this report could serve as the manual of the stereotypic checklist.

In the last study of this systematic series of reports, Berkson (1965) reported on four men from the same population previously studied. Because all the subjects engaged in stereotyped behavior, two medications (Dexedrine and Seconal) were administered at two dosage levels. There were no significant effects found as a result of medication administration. The author commented that the lack of effect was probably due to the low dosages used.

DISCUS

A normative study of all the residents in a mental retardation facility was completed to develop Dyskinesia Identification System—Condensed User Scale (DISCUS), which contained 34 items (Sprague et al., 1984). Of the 519 residents, 177 were rated independently by pairs of raters (14 total raters). The interrater correlations varied from a low of .14 on the holokinetic item to a high of .81 on tonic tongue. The total score reliability correlation was higher at .78 than most single items. Stability data were obtained on the same rater who examined residents about 1 week apart. These stability correlations varied from a low of −.03 on blepharospasm and upper-lip tremor items to a high of .65 on tongue tremors. The total score stability correlation was .77. In another way of calculating reliability, the totals of the 5,562 item ratings were compared on two criteria: strict criterion of exact agreement between two independent raters and lenient criterion of up to one point difference. Under the strict criterion, 4,318 (77.6%) of the ratings were exactly the same, but 5,235 (94.1%) of the ratings met the lenient criterion. A withdrawal-of-medication study (Kalachnik et al., 1984) was conducted on 191 of the subjects from this facility, and significant increases on ratings of TD were obtained as a result of neuroleptic medication withdrawal.

A revision of the scale was undertaken (Sprague, White, Ullmann, & Kalachnik, 1984). It is worth noting that this is the only TD scale that has been revised as recommended by psychometric standard 3.18 listed previously. A total of 191 developmentally delayed institutional residents were studied using six quality-of-item indicators: (a) *assessability*, the number of residents who could be rated on an item divided by the total sample of residents; (b) *interrater reliability correlation*; (c) *stability correlation*; (d) *observability*, the percentage of the ratings that were not zero; (e) *item versus total score correlation*; and (f) *discriminability*, the magnitude of the *F* test for testing the significance of the difference between a group of residents ($n = 86$) who had their neuroleptic medication gradually reduced and terminated compared to a group of residents ($n = 51$) who were randomly selected to remain on their neuroleptic medication. To equate the metrics for these diverse quality-of-item indicators, *Z* scores were calculated, and the 15 items with the largest *Z* scores were retained while the remaining items were eliminated.

After revision of the scale, another reliability study was conducted with 148 developmentally delayed residents (Sprague, Kalachnik, & Slaw, 1989). As could be expected after the elimination of less reliable items, the reliability correlations were improved. The lowest reliability correlation for two independent raters was .42 on blinking, and the highest was .79 for toe movement. The total score reliability was quite acceptable at .92. Stability of the revised scale was assessed over a 2-week time period in which the same rater examined the resident a second time. The lowest stability correlation was .10 for tongue tremor, and the highest was .75 on retrocollis/torticollis. The total score reliability correlation was .92.

In a study by Kalachnik, Sprague, and Slaw (1988), 263 people were trained in 14 workshops in five different states to use DISCUS (Sprague et al., 1984). The institutionalized people included veterans and developmentally disabled, mentally ill, and geriatric populations. Prior to the classroom part of the training workshop, a videotape of selected patients was shown and participants were asked to rate the videotape. After about 7 hours of classroom instruction and viewing of other videotapes, the test videotape was shown again, and the participants rated the videotape a second time. The basic data were the difference score (trainee rating minus criterion rating—a metric that could be either positive or negative in value) between the pretest rating and the posttest rating. In addition, the trainees rated patients from the facility where the workshop was held, and a difference score was calculated between the trainees' rating and the rating of the instructor. A large significant effect of training was found ($F = 122.19$; $df = 2$; $p < .0001$). On the pretraining test, the largest difference score (on a 5-point scale from 0 to 4) was -0.9 on chewing and the smallest difference score was 0.1 on ankle flexion and -0.1 on puckering. The mean total score (sum of the 15 individual items) difference was 5.3. The posttest difference scores were smaller; the biggest difference of -0.8 was found on three items. The smallest difference score was 0.0 on blinking, retrocollis, and shoulder torsion. The total score difference was -2.3. However, the best results of training were observed on the rating of the patients themselves in contrast to videotapes. This is an important finding because it indicates a good generalization from videotapes to the clinical situation of rating patients. The largest difference was 0.2 on ankle flexion, and the smallest was 0.0 on grimace, tongue tremor, and toe movement. The mean total score difference for the patients, -0.2, was smaller than for the posttest videotape difference.

The institutional population of a large state was assessed in another study examining the reliability and validity of the DISCUS (Sprague & Kalachnik, 1991). Of the total population ($N = 7,471$), 2,822 psychiatric patients and 4,649 mentally retarded residents were examined (Sprague & Kalachnik, 1991). Some raters ($n = 62$) were directly trained by one of the authors. In an attempt to examine whether indirect training could successfully be accomplished, the author trained staff who in turn trained an additional 277 people to use DISCUS. There was no significant difference in the scores of the raters receiving the two kinds of training (direct instruction by the author vs. indirect instruction by other trainers; $t = 1.06$; $df = 7,575$). A total of 277 psychiatric patients were independently rated by pairs of raters from a pool of 92 people trained in this study. The lowest reliability correlation was .45 for pill rolling and the highest correlation was .91 for retrocollis/torticollis. The total score reliability correlation was .92. For the 407 developmentally disabled individuals who were rated independently by pairs of raters from a pool of 128 trained in this study, the lowest reliability correlation was .57 for pill rolling, and the highest was .97 for shoulder/hip torsion. The total score correlation was .91.

Validity was assessed in this large sample; 108 physician-diagnosed TD participants were compared to a cohort of 108 subjects who were matched on sex, age, and neuroleptic medication status. The mean total score (8.0) of the physician-diagnosed TD group was significantly larger ($f = 39.87$; $df = 1, 24$; $p < .0001$) than the mean total score (3.4) of the cohort nondiagnosed group.

A different type of validity indicator was used in a study based on kinematic measures of finger tremor and postural stability or balance (Sprague, Korach, van Emmerik, & Newell, 1993). Finger tremor was measured by a lightweight accelerometer, which was attached to the index finger. Postural stability was measured on a force platform that indicated the postural sway of the residents. These recoding devices produced numerous measures. Developmentally delayed residents of a facility ($N = 36$) were included in an experiment using dynamic movement measures, which were compared to four selected items of the DISCUS. These four items (finger tremor, athetoid/myokymic finger–wrist–arm, pill rolling, and toe movement) were selected because they seemed most likely to correlate with the kinds of kinematic measures being taken. Because there was a large number of correlations obtained between the kinematic measures and the DISCUS items, only the pattern of correlations will be discussed as a validity indicator. On the DISCUS items that indicated some kind of rhythmic movement, patterns of significant correlations were found. Of the 16 finger-tremor measures, 8 significantly correlated with the tongue tremor item, and 0 correlated with the athetoid/myokymic item; 7 correlated with the pill-rolling item; and 0 correlated with the total score. On the 24 measures of postural balance, 0 correlated with tongue tremor, 0 with athetoid/myokymic, 0 with pill rolling, 6 with toe movement, and 8 with the total score.

Simpson Tardive Dyskinesia Scale

Albus et al. (1985) examined 36 male chronic schizophrenic patients using the Simpson Scale. In addition, the Brief Psychiatric Rating Scale was used and computed tomography (CT) scans were obtained. A significant correlation ($r = .54$) was found between the severity of TD and sulci enlargement.

Firth and Ardern (1985) examined 10 chronic schizophrenic patients using the Abbreviated Rockland Rating Scale. A clinical rater examined the patients and gave them a score, and then the patients were videotaped. After 6 months, the clinical rater and another rater again rated the videotapes. A total of 100 ratings were obtained. Percentage agreement was calculated on whether a symptom was present or absent, and there was 75% agreement between the clinician and other raters. When movement was present, 91% agreement was reached.

As described previously in the review of the AIMS literature, Gardos et al., (1983) also used the Simpson Scale over the 3-year study, which can be interpreted as an indication of the stability of the scale. All three measures increased on the Simpson Scale. Two of the mean increases were significant: 1.21 for restlessness and 1.87 for choreoathetosis.

Although the study (Izumi et al., 1986) involved treatment with medication to reduce TD symptoms, it does provide some 4-week stability data on the Simpson Scale. Japanese psychiatric patients ($N = 11$) were treated for 4 weeks with meclofenoxate at a dosage up to 1,200 mg/day. They were rated daily by one of the authors and examined weekly by that author and another author using the Simpson Scale. The medication resulted in a significant decrease ($p < .02$), on a statistical test that was not described, in 7 of the 11 patients. One piece of validating evidence, electromyographic recording, indicated that one patient showed a clear reduction in activity in five different muscles.

The Richardson and Craig (1982) study of the AIMS and Simpson has already been discussed previously with correlations between the items varying from a low of .10 to a high of .98. The Richardson et al. (1986) study, also reviewed previously, indicated reliability on the Simpson Scale for 25 subjects and two raters; reported Kappas varied from a low of .63 to a high of .74.

Simpson, Lee, Zoubok, and Gardos (1979) developed the Tardive Dyskinesia Rating Scale and a shorter version termed the Abbreviated Dyskinesia Scale. Reliability data were presented on 34 items for two raters who independently rated 26 patients. The item reliability correlations varied from a low of .55 for choreoathetoid tongue to .99 for grimacing. The total score reliability correlations was .98. Subsequently, 23 live patients and 9 videotapes were rated by nine raters. "The average pair-wide [sic] interrater reliability" (p. 173) was .79 to .99 for live patients and .87 to .91 for videotapes. The problem with the second set of data is that it is uncertain what is meant by "average" correlations; the authors do not give the precise details of how the correlations were calculated. As mentioned before, if the correlations were calculated by arithmetic averages, the data are misleading.

Sct. Hans Rating Scale

In this review, only one study (Hoffman, Labs, & Casey, 1987) could be found that gave some psychometric data on the Sct. Hans Rating Scale for Extrapyramidal Syndromes (Gerlach, 1979). In a study of 21 Veterans Administration patients, 10 of whom with diagnosed TD, a battery of tests was administered including Schedule for Affective Disorders and Schizophrenia—Lifetime Version, AIMS, Sct. Hans, CT scans, neuropsychological tests, and a treatment history. Multiple regression techniques were obtained to examine relationships among the battery of variables. No significant correlations were found between the AIMS and other tests including the Sct. Hans.

CONCLUSION

The standards for behavioral and psychological assessments (AERA et al., 1985) were reviewed, and 21 were selected that seem appropriate for instruments developed to assess abnormal movements. It was clear from the present review that none of the current instruments meet these ideal standards, and most of the widely used instruments are quite inadequate when measured against these psychometric standards. This indicates that the study of abnormal movements has generally paid little attention to the basic aspects of measuring symptoms, which is the beginning bedrock of any science undertaking a study of a disorder. It is unclear why the field has ignored this important aspect of developing sound measurements. It is speculated that the field has been so engrossed with clinical problems that basic properties of measurement often have been overlooked. This is most unfortunate because it has been repeatedly demonstrated in other fields that progress can be most rapidly made when proper attention is paid to accurate measurement.

It is quite surprising that only one of the scales (DISCUS) has been revised, although the first, AIMS, was published 18 years ago. On the other hand, considering that such little consideration has been given to the psychometric properties of these scales, perhaps the data needed for revision simply have not been collected by most of the scale developers and researchers.

Another revealing aspect of this review is that so little attention has been paid to training of raters to use these scales. The tacit assumption seems to be that if a person has some professional experience in the area, that person can automatically use these instruments without training. It should be apparent to most knowledgeable researchers that such an assumption is unlikely to be true. Our project on the DISCUS has shown in a clear manner that this assumption is not valid.[3] Training is even more important when direct care staff are used to rate patients. Furthermore, with the emphasis on cost-containment in medical treatment, it is even more likely that direct care staff will be expected to do the ratings because their salaries are generally lower than those of more highly trained medical personnel.

Another aspect of training that has been generally overlooked is whether training procedures can be developed that will enable people other than the developers of the scale or their close associates to train

---

[3]Kalachnik and Sprague (1994) studied 122 physicians, 82 pharmacists, and 78 psychologists for a total of 282 professionals using pretest and posttests as an indicator of the professionals' initial rating ability. None of the groups were significantly different at the pretest, and all the groups significantly improved with training.

raters. Although several studies have used videotapes to train colleagues at the same facility, only one study has systematically investigated training staff as a second generation of trainers and assessed the capability of the raters trained by them (Sprague & Kalachnik, 1991). State and federal government regulations indicate the importance of monitoring the side effects of neuroleptic medication. Then rational research must be conducted and training procedures will be needed for the large numbers of raters in facilities where neuroleptic medication may be used.

Finally, there are recent methodological developments that could be quite useful to improving the assessment of TD. In an excellent article about the usefulness of signal detection theory to the perplexing problem of diagnosis in psychiatry, Hsiao, Bartko, and Potter (1989) show the potential value of a new quantity—the receive operating characteristic—in improving diagnosis. They discuss the value of this technique for setting a cutoff score, which determines the *sensitivity* (true positive rate) and the *specificity* (false positive rate) of an instrument. In a technique arising from the interaction of neuroscience research and software development, Cohen, Sudhalter, Landon-Jimenez, and Keogh (1993) show the potential for neural network software to improve the accuracy and guide the theoretical development of diagnosis in the behavioral sciences and psychiatry. It is expected that such methodological advances will be used in the future to improve TD ratings.

REFERENCES

Ahrens, T. N., Sramek, J. J., Herrera, J. M., Jewett, C. M., & Alcorn, V. E. (1988). Pharmacy-based screening program for tardive dyskinesia. *Drug Intelligence and Clinical Pharmacy, 22,* 205–208.

Albus, M., Naber, D., Muller-Spahn, F., Douillet, P., Reinerthofer, T., & Ackenheil, M. (1985). Tardive dyskinesia: Relation to computer-tomographic, endocrine, and psychopathological variables. *Biological Psychiatry, 20,* 1082–1089.

American Educational Research Association, American Psychological Association, & National Council on Measurement in Education. (1985). *Standards for educational and psychological testing.* Washington, DC: American Psychological Association.

American Psychiatric Association. (1979). *Tardive dyskinesia.* Washington, DC: Author.

American Psychiatric Association. (1992). *Tardive dyskinesia: A task force report of the American Psychiatric Association.* Washington, DC: Author.

Barnes, T. R. E., Kidger, T., & Gore, S. M. (1983). Tardive dyskinesia: A 3-year follow-up study. *Psychological Medicine, 13,* 71–81.

Barnes, T. R. E., Rossor, M., & Trauer, T. (1983). A comparison of purposeless movements in psychiatric patients treated with antipsychotic drugs and normal individuals. *Journal of Neurology, Neurosurgery, and Psychiatry, 46,* 540–546.

Barnes, T. R. E., & Trauer, T. (1982). Reliability and validity of a tardive dyskinesia videotape rating technique. *British Journal of Psychiatry, 140,* 508–515.

Bergen, J. A., Griffiths, D. A., Rey, J. M., & Beumont, P. J. V. (1984). Tardive dyskinesia: Fluctuating patient or fluctuating rater. *British Journal of Psychiatry, 144,* 498–502.

Berkson, G. (1964). Stereotyped movements of mental defectives: V. Ward behavior and its relation to an experimental task. *American Journal of Mental Deficiency, 69,* 253–264.

Berkson, G. (1965). Stereotyped movements of mental defectives: VI. No effect of amphetamine or a barbiturate. *Perceptual and Motor Skills, 21,* 698.

Berkson, G., & Davenport, R. K. (1962). Stereotyped movements of mental defectives. *American Journal of Mental Deficiency, 66,* 849–852.

Berkson, G., & Mason, W. A. (1963). Stereotyped movements of mental defectives: III. Situation effects. *American Journal of Mental Deficiency, 68,* 409–412.

Berkson, G., & Mason, W. A. (1964). Stereotyped movements of mental defectives: IV. The effects of toys and the character of the acts. *American Journal of Mental Deficiency, 68,* 511–524.

Campbell, M., & Deutsch, S. I. (1985). Neuroleptics in children. In G. Burrows, T. R. Norman, & B. Davies (Eds.), *Antipsychotics* (pp. 213–238). Amsterdam: Elsevier.

Cohen, J., & Cohen, P. (1975). *Applied multiple regression/correlation analysis for the behavioral sciences.* Hillsdale, NJ: Lawrence Erlbaum Associates.

Cohen, I. L., Sudhalter, V., Landon-Jimenez, D., & Keogh, M. (1993). A neural network approach to the classification of autism. *Journal of Autism and Developmental Disorders, 23,* 443–466.

Davenport, R. K., & Berkson, G. (1963). Stereotyped movements of mental defectives: II. Effects of novel objects. *American Journal of Mental Deficiency, 67,* 879–882.

Firth, W. R., & Ardern, M. H. (1985). Measuring abnormal movement in tardive dyskinesia: A pilot study. *British Journal of Psychiatry, 147,* 723–726.

Gardos, G., & Cole, J. O. (1980). Problems in the assessment of tardive dyskinesia. In W. E. Fann, R. C. Smith, & J. M. Davis (Eds.), *Tardive dyskinesia: Research and treatment* (pp. 201–214). New York: Spectrum.

Gardos, G., Cole, J. O., & La Brie, R. (1977). The assessment of tardive dyskinesia. *Archives of General Psychiatry, 34,* 1206–1212.

Gardos, G., Perenyi, A., Cole, J. O., Samu, I., & Kallos, M. (1983). Tardive dyskinesia: Changes after three years. *Journal of Clinical Psychopharmacology, 3,* 315–318.

Gerlach, J. (1979). Tardive dyskinesia. *Danish Medical Bulletin, 26,* 206–245.

Germer, C. K., Seraydarian, L., & McBrearty, J. F. (1984). Training hospital clinicians to diagnose tardive dyskinesia. *Hospital and Community Psychiatry, 35,* 769–770, 783.

Guy, W. (1976). *ECDEU assessment manual for psychopharmacology* (DHEW Pub. No. ADM 76-338). Washington, DC: U.S. Government Printing Office.

Guy, W., Ban, T. A., & Wilson, W. H. (1985). An international survey of tardive dyskinesia. *Progress in Neuro-Psychopharmacology & Biological Psychiatry, 9,* 401–405.

Hoffman, W. F., Labs, S. M., & Casey, D. E. (1987). Neuroleptic-induced Parkinsonism in older schizophrenics. *Biological Psychiatry, 22,* 427–434.

Hsiao, J. K., Bartko, J. J., & Potter, W. Z. (1989). Diagnosing diagnoses. *Archives of General Psychiatry, 46,* 664–667.

Izumi, K., Tominaga, H., Koja, T., Nomoto, M., Shimizu, T., Sonoda, H., Imamura, K., Igata, A., & Fukuda, T. (1986). Meclofenoxate therapy in tardive dyskinesia: A preliminary report. *Biological Psychiatry, 21,* 151–160.

Jeste, D. V., & Wyatt, R. J. (1982). *Understanding and treating tardive dyskinesia.* New York: Guilford Press.

Kalachnik, J. E., Harder, S. R., Kidd-Nielsen, P., Errickson, E., Doebler, M., & Sprague, R. L. (1984). Persistent tardive dyskinesia in randomly assigned neuroleptic reduction, neuroleptic nonreduction, and no-neuroleptic history groups: Preliminary results. *Psychopharmacology Bulletin, 20,* 27–32.

Kalachnik, J. E., & Sprague, R. L. (1994). How well do physicians, pharmacists and psychologists assess tardive dyskinesia movements? *Annals of Pharmacotherapy,* *28,* 185–190.

Kalachnik, J. E., Sprague, R. L., & Slaw, K. M. (1988). Training clinical personnel to assess for tardive dyskinesia. *Progress in Neuro-Psychopharmacology and Biological Psychiatry, 12,* 749–762.

Lane, R. D., Glazer, W. M., Hansen, T. E., Berman, W. H., & Kramer, S. I. (1985). Assessment of tardive dyskinesia using the Abnormal Involuntary Movement Scale. *Journal of Nervous and Mental Disease, 173,* 353–357.

Richardson, M. A., & Craig, T. J. (1982). Tardive dyskinesia: Inter- and intra-rating scale comparisons. *Psychopharmacology Bulletin, 18,* 4–6.

Richardson, M. A., Haugland, M. A., Pass, R., & Craig, T. J. (1986). The prevalence of tardive dyskinesia in a mentally retarded population. *Psychopharmacology Bulletin, 22,* 243–249.

Schooler, N. R., & Kane, J. M. (1982). Research diagnoses for tardive dyskinesia. *Archives of General Psychiatry, 39,* 486–487.

Simpson, G. M., Lee, J. H., Zoubok, B., & Gardos, G. (1979). A rating scale for tardive dyskinesia. *Psychopharmacology, 64,* 171–179.

Simpson, G. M., & Singh, H. (1988). Tardive dyskinesia rating scales. *L'Encéphale, XIV,* 175–182.

Smith, J. M., Kucharski, L. T., Eblen, C., Knutsen, E., & Linn, C. (1979). An assessment of tardive dyskinesia in schizophrenic outpatients. *Psychopharmacology, 64,* 99–104.

Smith, J. M., Kucharski, L. T., Oswald, W. T., & Waterman, L. J. (1979). A systematic investigation of tardive dyskinesia in inpatients. *American Journal of Psychiatry, 136,* 918–922.

Sprague, R. L. (1985, November). *Relying on psychotropic drugs to obtain normalization: Some abnormalization outcomes.* Paper presented at the meeting of the Conference on Abnormal Involuntary Movements in the Developmentally Disabled, Sonoma, CA.

Sprague, R. L. (1986, June). *Psychometric aspects of evaluation and future technology of assessment.* Paper presented at the meeting of the International Conference on Mental Health Technology, Vancouver, BC.

Sprague, R. L. (1988, August). *Issues in the use of psychotropic medication with mentally retarded people.* Paper presented at the meeting of the American Psychological Association, Atlanta, GA.

Sprague, R. L., & Kalachnik, J. E. (1991). Reliability, validity, and a total score cutoff for the Dyskinesia Identification System: Condensed User Scale (DISCUS) with mentally ill and mentally retarded populations. *Psychopharmacology Bulletin, 27,* 51–58.

Sprague, R. L., Kalachnik, J. E., Breuning, S. E., Davis, V. J., Ullmann, R. K., Cullari, S., Davidson, N. A., Ferguson, D. G., & Hoffner, B. A. (1984). The Dyskinesia Identification System-Coldwater (DIS-Co): A tardive dyskinesia rating scale for the developmentally disabled. *Psychopharmacology Bulletin, 20,* 328–338.

Sprague, R. L., Kalachnik, J. E., & Slaw, K. M. (1989). Psychometric properties of the Dyskinesia Identification System: Condensed User Scale (DISCUS). *Mental Retardation, 27,* 141–148.

Sprague, R. L., Korach, M. S., van Emmerik, R. E. A., & Newell, K. M. (1993). Correlation between kinematic and rating scale measures of tardive dyskinesia in a developmentally disabled population. *Journal of Nervous and Mental Disease, 181,* 42–47.

Sprague, R. L., White, D., Ullmann, R. K., & Kalachnik, J. E. (1984). Methods for selecting items in a tardive dyskinesia rating scale. *Psychopharmacology Bulletin, 20,* 339–345.

6

The Dynamics of Stereotypic Behaviors: Movement Variance and Invariance in the Classification of Movement Disorders

Karl M. Newell

THE DYNAMICS OF STEREOTYPIC BEHAVIORS

S tereotypic behaviors are commonplace in a variety of population segments, but they are particularly apparent in the institutionalized developmentally disabled (Baumeister & Forehand, 1973; Berkson, 1967;
Lewis & Baumeister, 1982). Under any definition, stereotypy is viewed as
a limitation or problem of sensorimotor system control. Stereotypic behavior is poorly understood at all levels of brain–behavior analysis, although descriptively most definitions of stereotypy converge to embrace
terms or concepts such as excessive repetition of movement, minimal
movement variability, and movement sequences inappropriate to the context (cf. Berkson, 1983; Cooper & Dourish, 1990; Mason, 1991).

Inherent in the definitions of stereotypy is the notion that there are
some distinguishing features of the movement dynamics when stereotypic
and normal movement sequences are contrasted (Berkson & Gallagher,

The preparation of this chapter was supported in part by grant HD21212 from the National Institutes of
Health. Alex Antoniou, Richard van Emmerik, Young Ko, and Sam Slobounov helped with some of the
data analysis reported here. My colleague Robert Sprague has been instrumental in the ongoing development of this research program.

1986). In spite of the various claims, however, there has been no formal basis advanced to distinguish the movement dynamics of stereotypies from the dynamics of other categories of action. Indeed, there has been very little direct study of the dynamics of the postures and movements commonly labeled as stereotypic.

In this chapter, I provide a preliminary outline of the possible distinguishing movement properties of stereotypic behaviors. A key issue to be examined is whether there are unique features to the movement dynamics of stereotypies, in contrast to other movement categories. Subsidiary questions include: (a) What movement properties distinguish stereotypies from normal movements? and (b) What movement properties are invariant in stereotypic behaviors? The outcome of this approach to the study of stereotypies should shed some light on the question of whether movement analysis can contribute to the characterization of stereotypies and the identification of the unique movement properties of stereotypic behaviors.

The program of research drawn on here in the discussion of stereotypic behaviors is exemplified through data analysis of the dynamics of the stereotypic movements associated with tardive dyskinesia (Newell & Sprague, 1990; Newell, van Emmerik, Lee, & Sprague, 1993; Sprague & Newell, 1987). *Tardive dyskinesia* is that movement disorder syndrome that is reflected by the abnormal movements associated with prolonged regimens of neuroleptic medication (American Psychiatric Association [APA], 1980; Kalachnik, 1984). The abnormal movements of tardive dyskinesia are particularly prevalent in the peripheral effector systems such as the lips, tongue, fingers, and toes, but the excessive abnormal movements of tardive dyskinesia can be identified in a wide range of muscle groups and movement forms. The movement analysis approach to stereotypic behaviors outlined here also provides the potential answer to the long-standing debate about what, if any, are the distinguishing features of nondrug-induced institutionalized stereotypies of the developmentally disabled and the stereotypies of the tardive dyskinetic developmentally disabled.

Variance and Invariance in Stereotypic Movement Sequences

Most contemporary theoretical positions in motor control and skill acquisition attempt to account for the variance or invariance evident in movement sequences. The degree of validity inherent in the operational interpretation of the respective variance and invariance constructs, however, varies from one theoretical approach to another. A particular problem has been the definition of variance and invariance in motor control. Given that there is *always* variability in some aspect or another of the kinematics and kinetics of movement sequences from trial to trial, it has been natural to ask, no matter what the theoretical orientation, how little variability is allowable for a movement sequence to still be defined as invariant? Or, the question can be turned around to consider the complementary issue of how much variability must exist in the movement sequence before a given movement property is classified as variable.

The degree of variability inherent in the production of movement sequences has a significant place in determining the categories of action or skill qualities of the performer, including stereotypic behaviors (Newell et al., 1993). However, there are many possible movement parameters that can be analyzed in examinations of the variability of the dynamics of movement sequences. In the study of stereotypic behaviors, it seems reasonable to ask, given the emphasis on movement invariance, what properties of the stereotypic movement dynamics are invariant? Berkson and Gallagher (1986) approached this problem by suggesting that it was the topographic properties of the movement sequence that were invariant and that defined a given stereotypy. The notion of topography emphasizes the detailed description of, in this context, the stereotypic movement sequence; but the concept implies that all points of the field of the movement dynamics under consideration need to be mapped or analyzed. In short, the topographical concept does not help distinguish the variant and invariant features of movement sequences (Newell, 1986).

The approach that I have developed to considering the invariant properties of stereotypic behaviors draws on some of the ideas developed in the visual perception of biological motion (Cutting & Proffitt, 1982; Johannson, von Hofsten, & Jansson, 1980). In this view, the dynamics of biological motion can be partitioned into the three categories of absolute, relative, and common motion. I have suggested that the identification of movement action categories is based on a unique set of relative motion properties of the torso and limbs (Newell, 1985). In this view, each stereotypic behavior has a certain set of unique relative motions that define the occurrence (or lack thereof) of a given movement sequence or stereotypy. The form of movement behavior may be operationalized through determining the set of the relative motions of the body segments.

Thus, the invariant properties of the stereotypic behaviors are those relative motion properties that afford the perception and labeling of that activity. Interestingly, the invariant movement properties reflect nominal categories of unique relative motions that are drawn from the continuous ratio scale of the kinematics of the torso and limb segments. It is the unique set of the relative motions of the movement dynamics that are the invariant properties of stereotypic behaviors and other action categories. The perception of constancy in the variability of the dynamics of the relative motions is assumed to be based on the same principles as those from the perception of constancy when observations of more static forms are made as, for example, in the perception of the letter *a* in a variety of styles of handwriting.

The variance in stereotypic movement sequences from repetition to repetition tends to be primarily in the absolute properties of the movement dynamics. That is, the absolute motions of the body segments in space and time tend to vary to some greater or lesser degree from repetition to repetition of the stereotypy. This variance of the discrete movement spatial and temporal properties can be calculated by traditional statistical procedures (e.g., standard deviation) and analyzed as a function of population group, action category, and so on. The variance of the spatial measures is determined at a particular time, and the variance of the temporal measures is determined at a particular place. When the variance of movement is discussed in motor control it is typically in relation to these particular discrete absolute movement properties. The underlying assumption of most traditional views of movement control is that the variability is a reflection of some limitation or problem in system control (cf. Newell & Corcos, 1993).

Another way of viewing this analysis of movement properties is that the collective of discrete movement kinematics provides to the observer a dynamic geometry to the movement sequence. This geometry is, in essence, what is often referred to, particularly in the movement arts, as the movement *form*. The qualitative properties of this dynamic geometry are quite robust—a feature that affords perceptual constancy of motion in the face of considerable change in the absolute values of the discrete movement properties. The quantitative properties of the movement kinematics can, however, exhibit considerable variability from trial to trial. The degree of this variability in the discrete movement properties is often taken as an index of the skill of the individual.

A consideration of the absolute, common, and relative properties of the kinematics of human movement provides a framework to distinguish the invariant and variant properties of movement. It is proposed here that this framework to movement analysis also provides a basis to examine the invariant and variant properties of stereotypic behaviors (see also Newell, 1985, 1986). In particular, the framework provides a basis to answer the question regarding *what* it is about stereotypic behaviors that is invariant.

It follows from this analysis that it is the set of unique relative motions that defines a particular stereotypic behavior. Each stereotypic behavior has a particular set of relative motions that enables observers to identify this category of behavior within and between individuals. I have found no tests of this idea specifically directed at stereotypic behaviors, but there is some evidence for this notion in the identification of physical activities such as locomotion and throwing (Hoenkamp, 1978; Scully, 1987). Systematic perceptual judgment studies of stereotypic behaviors are required to test the generalization of this idea to stereotypic movements.

Given the application of this framework to the study of movement, it seems probable, however, that it is not toward the relative motions that observers are focused when they speak of invariance or low variability in stereotypic behaviors. It follows that the traditional proposal of invariance or low variability in stereotypies implicitly refers to the low variance of the absolute motion properties in contrast to what one might observe in other individuals performing the same activity. Or, maybe more generally, that the variance of the absolute motion of stereotypic behaviors is lower than observed in normal people performing other, possibly similar movement forms. Both possibilities (and maybe others) are open because the variance notion in stereotypy has not been addressed specifically in relation to particular properties of the movement dynamics.

In summary, the concept of invariance or lack of variability is essentially synonymous with the concept of stereotypic behavior. There is, however, no evidence to suggest that stereotypic behaviors are any more or less variable than the movements exhibited in other behavior categories. It is proposed here that the invariance concept has in practice been used primarily in relation to the notion of some order to the movement dynamics produced by the developmentally disabled, even when there is no apparent external goal to be achieved by the individual. However, this use of the term *invariance* is redundant because if one is observing order to repetitions of movement then there must be some property that is common or invariant to these repeated observations. In certain respects, the use of the term *invariance* with stereotypic is tautological. This conclusion still leaves open the possibility that the variance of the absolute movement properties of stereotypic behaviors is different from that exhibited by other population categories either in the same task or in other movement tasks, although there are no direct tests of this issue to date. In the next section, we describe some preliminary work from our laboratory that addresses the variance of the absolute motion properties of tardive dyskinetic, stereotypic behaviors.

Movement Variance as an Index of Stereotypy

Stereotypic behaviors have no apparent external goal to be realized by the individual. That is, if there is a goal to the stereotypic activity, it has been intrinsically determined either implicitly or explicitly by the subject. This distinguishing feature of stereotypic behaviors makes it impossible and inappropriate for an experimenter to try to elicit the behavior on cue. One can, however, increase the probability of stereotypic behaviors occurring by placing the individual into a particular environment that appears to support the elicitation of stereotypies. For example, it seems that stereotypic behaviors are highly prevalent in institutionalized developmentally disabled individuals when the subject is asked to wait unattended in a waiting room. On the other hand, certain individuals have particular environments in which they perform particular stereotypic behaviors.

This idiosyncratic feature of stereotypic behaviors increases the difficulty of examining in detail the dynamic properties of the stereotypic movement sequence. In short, the movement-measuring device must not be obtrusive to the contextual setting. This leaves videotape analysis of stereotypic movements as perhaps the most useful instrument for recording the movement sequences of stereotypies. However, a kinematic analysis of stereotypic behaviors with videotape requires that the recording follow a certain set of minimal biomechanical signal processing principles (Winter, 1990).

Recently, my colleagues and I have made a preliminary analysis of the variability of facial stereotypies in developmentally disabled tardive dyskinetic subjects (Sprague, van Emmerik, Slobounov, & Newell, in press). We have analyzed both lip and tongue stereotypic movements in terms of their kinematic variability within a repetitive movement sequence. The determination that the movement sequence to be analyzed was a stereotypy was made by experienced observers. We have also analyzed the kinematic variability of normal subjects producing preferred lip and tongue repetitive motion sequences that mimicked the movement pattern of the stereotypy so as to provide a normal-subject data set for contrast with the stereotypic movements. Lip and tongue repetitive motions involve few joint space degrees of freedom, and normal subjects can produce a rhythmic motion that appears by eye to mimic the form produced by the stereotypic action.

This comparison between stereotypic and normal movement variability is not a direct test of movement variability under the same task constraints, but it provides a first test of the relative variability of stereotypic motions and those of normal subjects mimicking a stereotypic motion. One can argue that the goal of the two groups of subjects is different because the goal of the subject producing the stereotypy is unknown and, therefore, the experimental contrast is not a direct test of the relative variability. However, it is also worth noting that the stereotypic motion of the tardive dyskinetic patient is presumably a well-practiced activity whereas the normal subjects have had no practice in producing the repetitive lip and tongue motion sequences. Thus, there is also a negative bias in this test against the normal group, but this design feature in some ways adds to the merits of the test examining the relative variability of movements in tardive dyskinetic and normal subjects.

Our analyses were of developmentally disabled individuals who were diagnosed by clinical signs and by rating scale to have tardive dyskinesia (Sprague et al., in press). In all cases, subjects had a long history of neuroleptic medication, although the exact medication history was not known. As we could record the stereotypies only when they occurred, not all subjects produced all categories of the facial stereotypies studied, and not all produced a set number of trials of each type of stereotypy. We evaluated the stereotypic behaviors for the qualitative and quantitative properties of the movement kinematics that reflect the relative and absolute motion categories defined earlier.

Figure 1 shows the position–time movement profiles of the upper and lower lips for two subjects during the execution of a behavioral sequence defined as stereotypic. These movement profiles suggest a high degree of coupling between the positions over time of the upper and lower lips. A cross-correlation analysis of the upper and lower lip time-series revealed a relation of $r = .86$ and $r = .92$ for Figures 1A and 1B, respectively. The movement patterns shown in Figure 1 are typical of the lip stereotypies observed in tardive dyskinetic developmentally disabled subjects, although some subjects produced an antiphase lip relation rather than the in-phase lip relation shown here.

Figure 1 (facing page)

Sample upper and lower lip position over time in stereotypic profiles for two different tardive dyskinetic subjects. Video frame rate is 30 Hz—hence, each frame = 33.33 ms. Lip-motion unit is pixels; cc = cross-correlation.

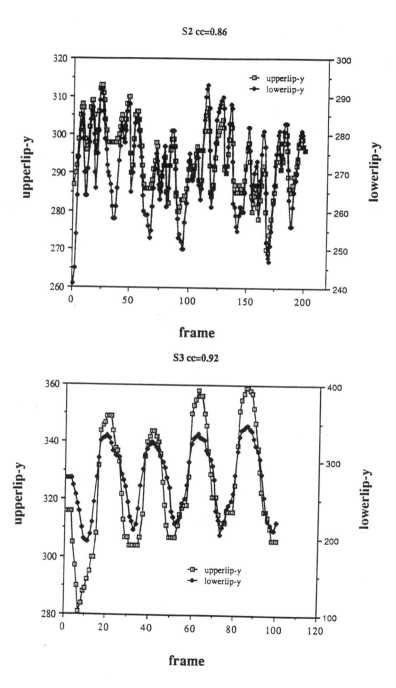

S2 cc=0.86

S3 cc=0.92

The form of each stereotypic motion was assessed through a pattern recognition analysis technique (Sparrow, Donovan, van Emmerik, & Barry, 1987). This analysis yields a coefficient value of 1.0, reflecting absolute similarity of movement form, and conversely a coefficient of 0.0, reflecting no coherence between the relative motion of the lip profiles. The pattern recognition coefficients ranged from 0.15 to 0.9 across the set of lip motion stereotypic trials examined. Thus, there were considerable individual differences in the variability of the movement form and yet this range of motion was still judged behaviorally as being reflective of a given stereotypic behavior. This finding is consistent with the perceptual constancy literature, which shows that considerable absolute variability in the properties of the observed form can still yield the same nominal perceptual judgment.

By contrast, the pattern coefficients for the normal subjects producing a preferred rhythmic lip motion ranged from .48 to .91. A sample kinematic lip motion time-series for a normal subject is shown in Figure 2. Thus, the range of movement-form coefficients is lower and the mean higher in the normal subjects, suggesting more stability in the movement form of the normal preferred rhythmic sequence. However, the normal subjects had a clear goal of reproducing a given movement form that may not have been the goal of the stereotypic subjects; therefore, this difference in stability of movement form may be due to differences in task constraints.

The variability of certain discrete kinematic properties of the lip cycles was also determined. The amplitude of motion, the peaks and troughs of the amplitude, and the timing properties of the rhythmic sequence were analyzed. On all kinematic parameters, the coefficient of variation of the stereotypic motions was higher than that of the respective parameter of the normal subjects producing a preferred rhythmic motion. This shows that the absolute variability of the stereotypic motions was higher than that of the rhythmic motions of the normal subjects. The coefficients of variation for the normal subjects (about .10 and below) were generally in the range recorded for other actions by normal healthy young adults (Newell, Carlton, & Hancock, 1984), whereas the tardive dyskinetic group

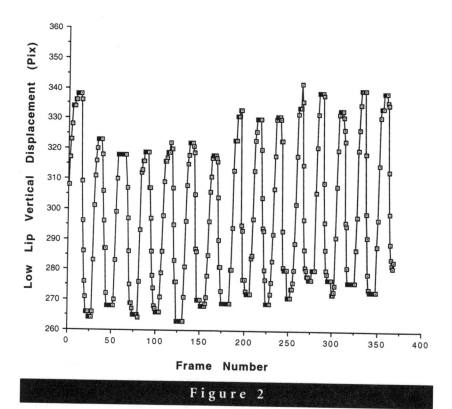

Figure 2

Sample upper lip motion of a normal subject producing a preferred rhythmic lip motion.

displayed relatively high absolute values (.10 to .40) to the coefficients of variation from the stereotypies.

The findings from these analyses of lip and tongue motions suggest that kinematic variability may not be the dimension that distinguishes stereotypic from normal movements. Indeed, the variability of stereotypic movements may not be generally lower than the variability of movements produced by normal subjects in a range of contextual circumstances. The task constraints for the two groups of subjects in our study could well be different (although this is difficult to determine either way), which militates against a direct test of the theoretical significance of this relative variability. On the other hand, the fact that normal subjects can produce such

125

low variability in unpracticed rhythmic movements represents an important baseline condition and leads to the proposal that movement variability is not the dimension to distinguish stereotypic behaviors. Further empirical tests are clearly required to examine the veracity of this claim.

The Structure of Movement Variability

The variability of movement is usually discussed in relation to the operational measure of the standard deviation of a given movement parameter. The standard deviation is taken as index of the variation inherent in the distribution of the respective movement parameter. The coefficient of variation (standard deviation divided by the mean) is a useful way to consider the relative variability of a given distribution. These measures allow one, as shown in the example of the variability of facial stereotypic movements, to consider the relative variability around different absolute mean values of the distribution.

The standard deviation of a distribution is, however, just one statistical property of a distribution. Moreover, the standard deviation does not provide any clues about the structure of the variability—it is simply a measure of the degree of variation inherent in a distribution. An additional and important measure of a distribution is an index of the structure of the trial-to-trial or sequence-to-sequence data that form the distribution. In discrete movement situations, this means having an index of the trial-to-trial relations of a given spatial or temporal outcome variable (Spray & Newell, 1986). In repetitive continuous motions, this implies some measure of the qualitative structure of the dynamics of the time-series (Newell et al., 1993).

In the last decade, there has been an increased use of techniques from nonlinear dynamics and dynamic systems theory to the analysis of biological motion (Beek, 1989; Garfinkel, 1983; Haken, Kelso, & Bunz, 1985; Kay, 1988; Saltzman & Kelso, 1987). A key focus in this approach is a consideration of the qualitative properties of the dynamics of motion and the attractor organization of the dynamics. Attractors, in the motor control domain, can be considered as building blocks for the field properties (collection of points) of the dynamics inherent in perceptual–motor work spaces (Kugler & Turvey, 1987; Newell, Kugler, van Emmerik, & McDonald, 1989). Attractors reflect equilibrium regions on which a set of different starting conditions in the state-space settles. There is a small set of distinct attractor types that exist across physical and biological systems, and there are measurement techniques available to determine these qualitative properties of the dynamics. A particularly useful measure is that of dimensionality, which, as the name implies, calculates the number of coordinates or degrees of freedom of the system that have produced the dynamic inherent in the time-series (Packard, Crutchfield, Farmer, & Shaw, 1980). Thus, this measure is particularly suited to be used in relation to the degrees of freedom problem in motor control (Bernstein, 1967; Kay, 1988). There are several difficulties inherent in determining the *absolute* dimensionality of a time-series, but there seems general agreement that this measure is useful in estimating the *relative* dimensionality of different time-series (Mayer-Kress, 1986; Rapp, Albana, & Mees, 1988).

In an ongoing study, my colleagues and I recently have applied the dimensionality measure to understand the structure inherent in the time-series of a whole-body postural dynamic (the center of pressure) and the finger tremor dynamic (acceleration profile) in individuals with diagnosed tardive dyskinesia. The purpose was to ascertain the relation between the qualitative structure of the stereotypic dynamic and the emergent movement variability of that dynamic as revealed in standard measures of variability, such as the standard deviation and the coefficient of variation. The working hypothesis from a motor-control and degrees-of-freedom perspective was that the variability in the standard discrete kinematic measures is inversely related to the dimensionality of the attractor supporting the respective action. I now provide some illustrative data from this ongoing work.

In our preliminary analysis of postural stability in developmentally disabled tardive dyskinetic subjects (Ko, van Emmerik, Sprague, & Newell, 1992), we found that approximately 38% of the trials showed a clear (to the eye of an observer) rhythmic pattern to the time-series of the center of pressure. In addition, and as expected, the variability of the center of pressure was greater in the tardive dyskinetic subjects than in the age-matched controls. In a subsequent analysis (Newell et al., 1993), we determined the dimensionality of the center of pressure on trials that were clearly rhythmic, on those that were not rhythmic in the tardive dyskinetic group, and in the apparently nonstructured center of pressure dynamics of the control group. Sample trials showing the center of pressure profile for these three groups are shown in Figure 3.

Our analysis revealed that on average the dimensionality was 1.30 for the rhythmic tardive dyskinesia group, 1.75 for the nonrhythmic tardive dyskinesia group, and 2.20 for the normal control group (Newell et al., 1993). This confirmed that the dimensionality of the center of pressure dynamics was higher in the normal control group, suggesting that the degrees of freedom regulated by normal subjects in the control of posture was also higher. Interestingly, the dimensionality measure distinguished between the tardive dyskinesia unstructured group and the normal control group, even though the movement dynamics of both groups appeared unstructured to the eye. The findings from this study suggest that the dimensionality measure may discriminate between dynamic conditions that are not discernible to the eye of observers and, therefore, could be useful as a diagnostic tool in the assessment of movement disorders.

We have also used the dimensionality measure to examine the structure inherent in the finger acceleration tremor of normal and tardive dyskinetic subjects (Newell, Gao, & Sprague, 1995). As one might expect, the degree and variability of motion of the finger tremor is greater in tardive dyskinetic than in normal subjects (van Emmerik, Sprague, & Newell, 1993). However, our preliminary analysis from Newell et al. (1995) also suggests that the dimensionality of finger tremor is lower in tardive dyskinetic subjects than in normal subjects. Figure 4 shows the mean dimensionality estimates for a developmentally disabled tardive dyskinetic group and an age-matched normal group. The mean dimensionality for

Figure 3 (facing page)

Sample center of pressure profiles over 10-s trials for three subjects: (a) normal subject, unstructured trial; (b) tardive dyskinetic subject, unstructured trial; and (c) tardive dyskinetic subject, rhythmic trial.

Scale 1.27

Y (cm)

X (cm)

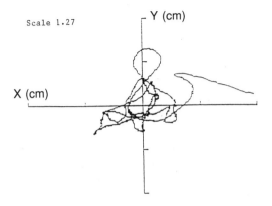

Scale 5.08

Y (cm)

X (cm)

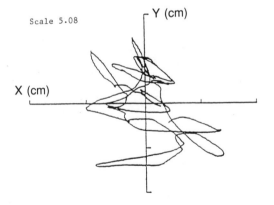

Scale 15.24

Y (cm)

X (cm)

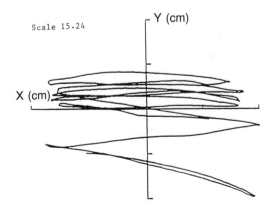

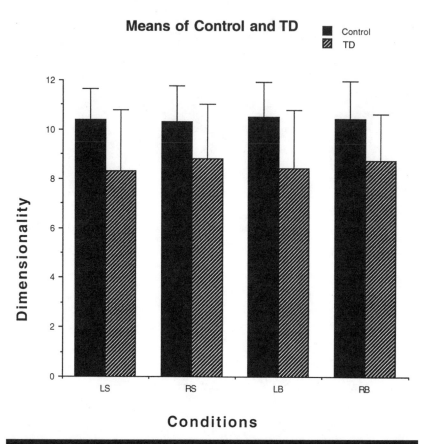

Means of Control and TD

■ Control
▨ TD

Dimensionality

Conditions

Figure 4

The dimensionality of finger tremor as a function of group (Control = Normal Subjects; TD = Tardive Dyskinetic Subjects) and finger task condition (LS = Left finger single; RS = Right finger single; LB = Left finger in the both fingers condition; RB = Right finger in the both fingers condition).

the tardive dyskinetic group was just over 8, but for the normal group was approximately 10. It was also the case that these estimates were essentially the same when index fingers were considered individually and when the fingers were examined in combination. The data also suggest that the structure of normal tremor is not stochastic, although clearly it has a high dimensionality. The dimensionality of finger tremor is higher than that of postural tremor, but the results are consistent across both postural tasks in showing reduced dimensionality in the tardive dyskinetic as opposed to the normal subjects.

In summary, the dimensionality measure appears to distinguish consistently between our tardive dyskinetic group and our normal age-matched control group. The general implication of our findings is that the dimensionality of the dynamics supporting whole-body posture and finger tremor is of a lower dimensionality in tardive dyskinetic subjects. In other words, the structure of the attractor dynamic supporting the postural tasks is more constrained in tardive dyskinetic subjects. This finding also suggests that the variability of discrete kinematic movement properties can be considered only in relation to the nature of attractor dynamic supporting the action. One cannot infer relative stability of a dynamic from the variability measure alone because different time-series may have different attractor equilibrium regions (Newell et al., 1993). Comparing the variability of movement across different attractor types as a basis to infer relative stability of, for example, posture is like comparing apples and oranges.

Variability and Degrees of Freedom

The discussed example of the relation between attractor organization of the movement dynamics and the resultant outcome variability in both stereotypic and normal movement demonstrates the degrees-of-freedom problem in motor control (Bernstein, 1967). It points to the need to consider movement dynamics not just at the joint space level, but also at an abstract control space level. Our data provide an example of the notion that the degrees of freedom to the attractor organization at the control space (perceptual–motor workspace) level will often be fewer than those evident at the joint space level (Kay, 1988; Newell et al., 1989; Saltzman & Kelso, 1987).

Our data also speak directly to the proposal that the performance (however it may be typically measured in a given task) is often inversely related to the degrees of freedom regulated in the perceptual–motor control space. In the whole-body postural example outlined previously, the dimensionality of the center of pressure dynamic was reduced as the variability on the behavioral level was increased. Thus, there is an inverse relation between the number of degrees of freedom regulated and the resultant performance. It may take practice for additional degrees of freedom to be introduced into the control space, but when they are, there is a related improvement in performance. This notion is counter to many intuitions and assumptions of the extant literature about the complexity of movement as viewed from the standpoint of the number of body segments involved in the coordination mode. It is also an empirical question as to what degree, if any, can subjects independently vary the dimensionality of the attractor dynamic supporting action and the variability of performance outcome.

The data from our studies also suggest that the reduction in the biomechanical degrees of freedom not only occurs in tasks where there are many degrees of freedom in the joint space to be regulated but, in addition, that the principles operate in the apparently oft-called simple single degree of freedom task of finger tremor. It appears that a prevailing consequence of tardive dyskinesia is a reduction in the degrees of freedom regulated at the control space level. One can also consider stereotypic actions in the same way and suggest that they are overconstrained in relation to the control exerted by normal subjects mimicking similar motions. This extra constraint on the motor system relates directly to the adaptability of the system. Indeed, it may well be that adaptability is a more useful distinguishing characteristic of stereotypic behavior than movement variability. I now pursue this issue briefly.

Stereotypy and Adaptability of Movement Dynamics

It is generally assumed that as the neuroleptic drug regimen continues over time, not only is the likelihood of the onset of tardive dyskinesia increased (APA, 1980; Kalachnik, 1984), but, in addition, the resultant stereotyped behavior becomes increasingly inflexible and unresponsive to environmental change (Cooper & Dourish, 1990). Even in institutionalized stereotypies, that is, in nondrug-induced stereotypic behaviors, it is assumed that as the strength of the stereotypy increases through continued practice, it is harder to modify the stereotypic behavior (Berkson, 1983). There are several independent but related facets, however, to this nonadaptive property of stereotypic behaviors.

The major view of the nonadaptive properties of stereotypic behavior relates to the enhanced difficulty in modifying the probability of the onset of the behavior. That is, it is difficult to change the likelihood of the occurrence of the behavior. Indeed, in tardive dyskinesia, the clinician has to consider the special circumstance of the fact that withdrawing the neuroleptic medication that caused the onset of stereotypic movements usually has the initial effect of increasing the probability and strength of the resultant abnormal movement sequences. There is still considerable debate about the degree to which tardive dyskinesia is reversible (Haag, Ruther, & Hippius, 1992). Thus, adaptability of the behavior in relation to the onset of its occurrence is a major concern with stereotypic behavior, particularly those stereotypic movements associated with tardive dyskinesia. In tardive dyskinesia, the ongoing considerations about the type of neuroleptic medication are based in part on their perceived effects on the adaptability of the abnormal movements.

Another aspect of the adaptability of stereotypic behaviors is the facility with which an individual may stop or move out of the respective behavior to engage in another action—one that may be related to either an external demand or an intrinsically determined goal on the part of the individual. The adaptability of the ongoing stereotypic behavior has not been studied adequately, in part because more emphasis has been given to the prevalence or initiation of stereotypic behaviors. The adaptability of ongoing stereotypic behaviors has been studied only in the context of their variability and, as was outlined previously, the empirical work even in this approach is limited. However, the relative facility of being able to switch out of a movement sequence is as much a part of behavioral adaptability as the facility of switching into a movement sequence.

The ease of probability of switching in and out of particular coordination modes (e.g., stereotypic behaviors) can be predicted on the basis or understanding of the structure of the attractor dynamics that are supporting the behaviors in question (Haken et al., 1985). One measure that can be used to investigate this phenomenon is the time it takes to switch into and out of a given coordination mode (Kelso, Scholtz, & Schoner, 1988). These relative switch times can be predicted a priori if one has characterized the structure of the attractor dynamics supporting the movement behavior in question. These kinds of switching-movement experiments could be conducted in the context of certain stereotypies.

Another facet of dynamic approaches to motor control is that they have begun to characterize where in the attractor region the subject is operating while being engaged in a particular activity. The emerging view is that skilled performers do not operate in the basin of the attractor equilibrium region, but rather operate at some distance away from this on a gradient of the dynamic to facilitate change or adaptability (Beek, 1989). This approach to motor control provides a formal basis to a long held viewpoint that skilled behavior is flexible and adaptable. Similar examinations could be made of stereotypic behaviors to determine if these movement sequences are more rigid to ongoing change than similar normal movements. A significant contribution of this approach to movement control is that it provides a principled rationale to the issue of adaptability of behavior.

The preceding analysis suggests that adaptability of stereotypic behaviors needs to be considered from both an initiation and a change of behavior perspective. Davis (1970) has shown in a preliminary analysis that the developmentally disabled were slow at switching out of a given stereotypic behavior. Nonadaptability or limited adaptability, as operationalized by a dynamic characterization of movement sequences, may prove to be a distinguishing feature of stereotypic behavior.

CONCLUSION

Although the availability of more data on the variability and stereotypy issue is desirable, the theoretical and empirical analyses presented here suggest that movement variability (or, more accurately, the lack of it) will not prove to be *the* (or even *a*) distinguishing feature of stereotypic behaviors. It does appear, however, that the qualitative characteristics of the dynamics of stereotypic behaviors may well be of a lower dimensionality than those of similar so-called normal movement patterns. This reduction in dimensionality of the perceptual–motor workspace in stereotypies also has the consequence of decreasing the adaptability of the system. The adaptive qualities of stereotypic movements and the normal movements, in general, of subjects who display stereotypies have not been a focus of systematic research. The analysis presented here, from a motor-control, degrees-of-freedom perspective, suggests that overconstraint on the system leads to reduced adaptability, which may well be a more distinguishing feature of stereotypies than reduced movement variability.

REFERENCES

American Psychiatric Association. (1980). *Task force report: Tardive dyskinesia.* Washington, DC: Author.

Baumeister, A. A., & Forehand, R. (1973). Stereotyped acts. In N. R. Ellis (Ed.), *International review of research in mental retardation.* (Vol. 6., pp. 55–96). New York: Academic Press.

Beek, P. (1989). *Juggling dynamics.* Amsterdam: Free University Press.

Berkson, G. (1967). Abnormal stereotyped motor acts. In J. Zubin & H. F. Hunt (Eds.), *Comparative psychopathology—Animal and human* (pp. 76–94). New York: Grune & Stratton.

Berkson, G. (1983). Repetitive stereotyped behaviors. *American Journal of Mental Deficiency, 88,* 239–246.

Berkson, G., & Gallagher, R. J. (1986). Control of feedback from abnormal stereotyped behaviors: I. In M. G. Wade (Ed.), *The development of coordination, control and skill in the mentally handicapped* (pp. 7–24). Amsterdam: North-Holland.

Bernstein, N. A. (1967). *The coordination and regulation of movements.* New York: Pergamon.

Cooper, S. J., & Dourish, C. T. (Eds.). (1990). *Neurobiology of stereotyped behavior.* Oxford, England: Clarendon Press.

Cutting, J. E., & Proffitt, D. R. (1982). The minimum principle and the perception of absolute, common, and relative motions. *Cognitive Psychology, 14,* 211–246.

Davis, K. V. (1970). *The effect of drugs on stereotyped and nonstereotyped operant behaviors in retardates.* Unpublished doctoral dissertation, University of Illinois.

Garfinkel, A. (1983). A mathematics for physiology. *American Journal of Physiology, 245*, R455–R466.

Grassberger, P., & Procaccia, I. (1983). Measuring the strangeness of strange attractors. *Physica, 9D*, 189–208.

Haag, H., Ruther, E., & Hippius, H. (1992). *Tardive dyskinesia.* Seattle: Hogrefe & Huber.

Haken, H., Kelso, J. A. S., & Bunz, H. (1985). A theoretical model of phase transitions in human hand movements. *Biological Cybernetics, 51*, 347–356.

Hoenkamp, E. (1978). Perceptual cues that determine the labeling of gait. *Journal of Human Movement Studies, 4*, 59–69.

Johansson, G., von Hofsten, C., & Jansson, G. (1980). Event perception. *Annual Review of Psychology, 31*, 27–63.

Kalachnik, J. E. (1984). Tardive dyskinesia and the mentally retarded: A review. In S. E. Bruening (Ed.), *Advances in mental retardation and developmental disabilities.* (Vol. 2, pp. 329–356). Greenwich, CT: JAI.

Kay, B. A. (1988). The dimensionality of movement trajectories and the degrees of freedom problem: A tutorial. *Human Movement Science, 7*, 343–364.

Kelso, J. A. S., Scholtz, J. P., & Schoner, G. (1988). Dynamics governs switching among patterns of coordination in biological movement. *Physics Letters A, 134*, 8–12.

Ko, Y. G., van Emmerik, R. E. A., Sprague, R. L., & Newell, K. M. (1992). Postural stability, tardive dyskinesia, and developmental disability. *Journal of Intellectual Disability Research, 36*, 309–323.

Kugler, P. N., & Turvey, M. T. (1987). *Information, natural law, and the self-assembly of rhythmic movement.* Hillsdale, NJ: Erlbaum.

Lewis, M. H., & Baumeister, A. A. (1982). Stereotyped mannerisms in mentally retarded persons: Animal models and theoretical analyses. In N. R. Ellis (Ed.), *International review of research in mental retardation.* (Vol. II, pp. 123–161). New York: Academic Press.

Mason, G. J. (1991). Stereotypies: A critical review. *Animal Behavior, 41*, 1015–1037.

Mayer-Kress, G. (Ed.). (1986). *Dimensions and entropies in chaotic systems.* New York: Springer-Verlag.

Newell, K. M. (1985). Coordination, control and skill. In D. Goodman, I. Franks, & R. Wilberg (Eds.), *Differing perspectives in motor control* (pp. 295–318). Amsterdam: North Holland.

Newell, K. M. (1986). Comments on coordination, control and skill papers. In

M. G. Wade (Ed.), *Motor skill acquisition of the mentally handicapped* (pp. 101–112). Amsterdam: North Holland.

Newell, K. M., Carlton, L. G., & Hancock, P. A. (1984). Kinetic analysis of response variability. *Psychological Bulletin, 96,* 133–151.

Newell, K. M., & Corcos, D. M. (1993). Issues in variability and motor control. In K. M. Newell & D. M. Corcos (Eds.), *Variability and motor control.* Champaign, IL: Human Kinetics.

Newell, K. M., Gao, F., & Sprague, R. L. (1995). The dynamics of finger tremor in tardive dyskinesia. *Chaos, 5,* 43–47.

Newell, K. M., Kugler, P. N., van Emmerik, R. E. A., & McDonald, P. V. (1989). Search strategies and the acquisition of coordination. In S. A. Wallace (Ed.), *Perspectives on the coordination of movement* (pp. 85–122). Amsterdam: North Holland.

Newell, K. M., & Sprague, R. L. (1990). Early diagnosis of tardive dyskinesia. In A. Vermeer (Ed.), *Motor development, adapted physical activities and mental retardation* (pp. 30–46). Amsterdam: North Holland.

Newell, K. M., van Emmerik, R. E. A., Lee, D., & Sprague, R. L. (1993). On postural stability and variability. *Gait & Posture, 4,* 225–230.

Packard, N. H., Crutchfield, J. D., Farmer, J. D., & Shaw, R. S. (1980). Geometry from a time series. *Physical Review Letters, 45,* 712–716.

Rapp, P. E., Albana, A. M., & Mees, A. I. (1988). Calculation of correlation dimension from experimental data: Progress and problems. In J. A. S. Kelso, A. J. Mandel, & M. F. Schlesinger (Eds.), *Dynamic patterns in complex systems* (pp. 191–205). Singapore: World Publishing.

Saltzman, E., & Kelso, J. A. S. (1987). Skilled action: A task dynamic approach. *Psychological Review, 94,* 84–106.

Scully, D. M. (1987). *Perception of biological motion.* Unpublished doctoral dissertation, University of Illinois at Urbana-Champaign.

Sparrow, W. A., Donovan, E., van Emmerik, R. E. A., & Barry, E. B. (1987). Using relative motion plots to measure change in intra-limb and inter-limb coordination. *Journal of Motor Behavior, 19,* 115–129.

Sprague, R. L., & Newell, K. M. (1987). Toward a movement control perspective of tardive dyskinesia. In H. Y. Meltzer (Ed.), *Psychopharmacology: The third generation of progress* (pp. 1233–1238). New York: Raven.

Sprague, R. L., van Emmerik, R. E. A., Slobounov, S. M., & Newell, K. M. (in press). Facial stereotypic movements and tardive dyskinesia in a developmentally disabled population. *American Journal of Mental Retardation.*

Spray, J. A., & Newell, K. M. (1986). Time series analysis of motor learning: KR versus no KR. *Human Movement Science, 5,* 59–74.

van Emmerik, R. E. A., Sprague, R. L., & Newell, K. M. (1993). Finger tremor and tardive dyskinesia. *Experimental and Clinical Psychopharmacology, 1,* 259–268.

Winter, D. A. (1990). *Biomechanics and motor control of human movement.* New York: Wiley.

7

Normal Infant Stereotypies: A Dynamic Systems Approach

Esther Thelen

Over a decade ago, I described a class of repetitive movements of the limbs, torso, head, or whole body in normally developing infants, which I called *rhythmical stereotypies* (Thelen, 1979). Many other authors had commented upon the unusual stereotyped banging, waving, rocking, shaking, and bouncing movements that appear as transient phases in normal infants, but are most often associated with severe mental or emotional pathologies, deprivation, or drug use (e.g., Hutt & Hutt, 1965; Kaufman & Levitt, 1965; Kravitz & Boehm, 1971; Lourie, 1949; Wolff, 1968). Indeed, Berkson (1967) had earlier suggested that pathological stereotyped behavior may well be fixations of or regressions to the normal, transient developmental stereotypies typical of the first year or so of life.

In this chapter, I propose that, whereas it may be difficult to find a real developmental continuity between the transient stereotypies of infancy to the rigid pathological movements of concern to mental health specialists, a common process underlies both. This is the tendency of neuromotor systems under undeveloped or impaired voluntary control to oscillate naturally. Secondarily, these natural oscillations may be appropriated by the organism for other goals: to explore the environment, communicate, or provide sensory stimulation in an impoverished environment.

I now have a detailed understanding of infant stereotypies at many levels of analysis, from descriptive behavior to fine measurements of the kinematics of the movements, the forces moving the limbs and segments, and the muscle patterns underlying these movements. My colleagues and I also know something about the developmental changes in these movements, especially in the transitions between rhythmical stereotypies and goal-corrected movements such as locomotion and reaching. By understanding how stereotypies emerge, and how they are controlled, are modulated, and later regress in normal infancy, insight may be gained into the brain–body–behavior–environment relations in these mysterious behaviors in other populations.

A NATURAL HISTORY OF NORMAL INFANT RHYTHMICAL STEREOTYPIES

Because previous interpretations of infant stereotypy were burdened with theory and light on data (Thelen, 1981b), I began my study of these movements with an intensive natural history phase: observations of normal infants in their homes to describe the form and context of rhythmical movements. I followed 20 normal infants every other week from age 4 weeks until 1 year. Each infant was observed for 1 hour, and observers coded all instances of rhythmical movements and their immediate contexts and simultaneously sampled the ongoing behavior of infant and caregiver (Thelen, 1979). This dual coding scheme resulted in developmental profiles of occurrences and frequencies of movement and, in addition, provided information on the immediate circumstances associated with particular stereotypy bouts.

A rich and detailed picture of these movements emerged from observations alone. First, it was evident that normal infants performed rhythmical movements of their limbs and body segments many times over the first year. (I recorded over 16,000 bouts of such movements.) Infants performed stereotyped and repetitive movements of both upper and lower limbs and of the whole body in every posture (Figures 1, 2, and 3). Such kicking, rocking, waving, banging, bouncing, and thumping movements were seen in all the infants and at around 6 months of age, when stereotypy rate was the highest, often accounted for 10% to 20% of the time of observation (Thelen, 1979).

The various movement types were not randomly distributed over all ages. Rather, they were specifically and strikingly associated with transitions between no voluntary control over the limb or body segment and adaptive and intentional control. Figure 4 summarizes the frequencies of rhythmical stereotypies for the sample as a function of age and the body group involved. What is notable is that most of these movements had a well-delineated time of both onset, peak, and decline, and that this developmental trajectory was coincident with emergent voluntary control. Thus, kicking the legs was most prevalent before locomotion, rocking appeared before crawling, waving the arms coincided with emergent reaching, banging came before good manipulatory control of the hand, and swaying peaked just as infants gained good standing control. Indeed, there was a significant correlation between the ages of onset of rhythmical stereotypies and selected motor milestones as measured by the Bayley Scales.

Infants also did not perform stereotyped movements at equal rates across all possible contexts of their daily life (Thelen, 1981a). Rather, particular eliciting situations at particular ages were more likely to trigger bouts of such movements. To normalize for the naturally differing amounts of time infants spend in particular behavioral contexts as they get older (older infants sleep and cry less, for instance), I created a ratio expressing the number of bouts of total stereotypy in a particular context at each observation divided by the estimate of time spent in that context obtained by our time-sampling data. These data are illustrated in Figure 5. Over the first year, more stereotypy was associated with nonalert states (crying, drowsing, but mostly fussing) than with other situations, but other eliciting contexts included social interactions with the caregiver, passive and active position changes, feeding, and handling objects.

This naturalistic study provided systematic empirical support to earlier

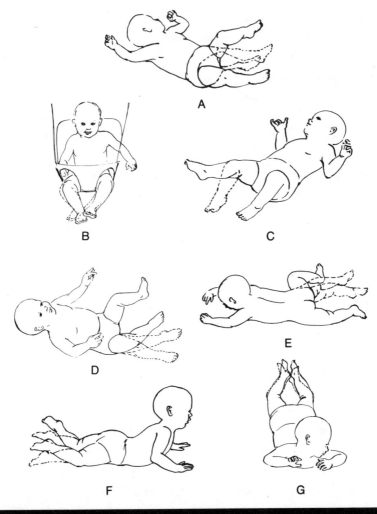

Figure 1

Rhythmical stereotypies of the legs. The individual drawings show: (A) alternate-leg kicking in supine; (B) foot rubbing; (C) single-leg kicking in supine; (D) single-leg kicking in supine with the leg rotated outward; (E) single-leg kicking in prone; (F) both-legs-together kicking; (G) both-legs-together kicking with the back strongly arched. From *Animal Behaviour, 27,* 619–715. Copyright 1979 by Academic Press. Reprinted with permission of the publisher.

suggestions that motor rhythmicities were a normal concomitant of maturation and were particularly evident in times of transition, when full voluntary control of an action was still emerging (Lourie, 1949). The developmental importance of these movements has recently been confirmed by

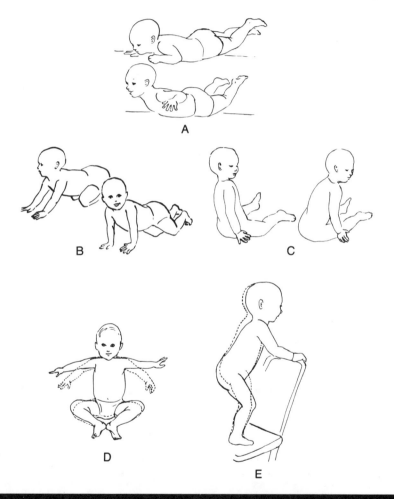

Figure 2

Rhythmical stereotypies of the whole torso. The individual drawings show: (A) arched-back rocking; (B) hands-and-knees rocking; (C) sit-rocking, sitting unsupported; (D) sit-bouncing, sitting unsupported; (E) stand-bouncing. From *Animal Behaviour, 27*, 619–715. Copyright 1979 by Academic Press. Reprinted with permission of the publisher.

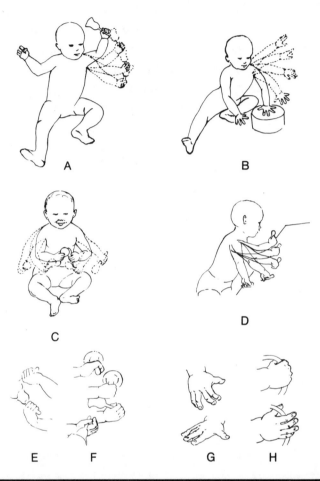

Figure 3

Rhythmical stereotypies of the arms, hands, and fingers. The individual drawings show: (A) arm waving with object; (B) arm banging against surface; (C) banging with both arms together with object; (D) arm sway; (E) hand flex; (F) hand rotate; (G) and (H) finger flex. From *Animal Behaviour, 27,* 699–715. Copyright 1979 by Academic Press. Reprinted with permission of the publisher.

a study comparing types and rates of stereotypy in motor-impaired, Down syndrome, and nondisabled children (MacLean, Ellis, Galbreath, Halpern, & Baumeister, 1991). These authors found that disabled subjects displayed a developmental course of rhythmic behaviors similar to that of nondisabled subjects when the data were expressed in terms of motor–age equivalence. However, the motor-impaired subjects performed significantly less rhythmic behavior per session than the other groups and proportionately more specific head movements.

Our naturalistic studies led to several conclusions about these distinctive movements. First, rhythmical stereotypies are expressions of the natural oscillations of the neuromotor system when voluntary control is becoming established. They are transitional behaviors in the sense that they are performed when infants have some level of control over

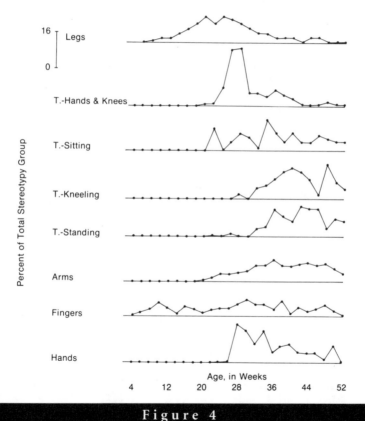

Figure 4

Frequencies of groups of rhythmical stereotypies during the first year. Frequencies have been expressed at each age as a percentage of the total bouts of that stereotypy group seen at that age. Vertical scale indicated at top left is the same for each horizontal axis. The data are pooled, $N = 20$. (T = Torso). From *Animal Behaviour*, *27*, 699–715. Copyright 1979 by Academic Press. Reprinted with permission of the publisher.

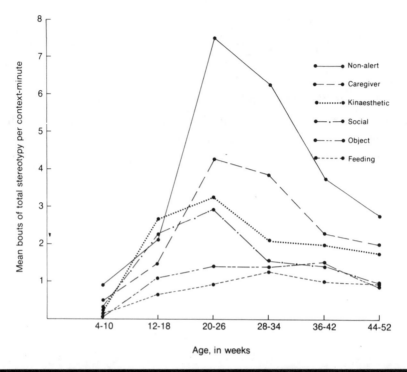

Figure 5

Mean bouts of stereotypy using legs, torso, and arms per context-minute in six infant states and eliciting contexts during the first year. From *Animal Behaviour, 29,* 3–11. Copyright 1981 by Academic Press. Reprinted with permission of the publisher.

the body parts involved—for example, when they assume a particular posture—but have not yet acquired the ability to adapt their actions to an intentional goal. Infants flap their arms before they can reach, rock before they crawl, and bounce before they walk. The movements are rhythmical because cyclicity is often a preferred temporal pattern in complex, dynamic systems under particular energetic configurations (see Thelen, Kelso, & Fogel, 1987). In dynamic terms, cyclicity is an attractor, an emergent pattern, that "pulls in" other possible coordinations. It is as though the infants, in the appropriate posture or context, wish to behave and thus activate the system, but in the absence of the appropriate goal-directed skill, express a pattern into which the system naturally falls—oscillation (Thelen, 1979). Thus, stereotypies were commonly seen when infants were excited or fussy—diffuse states in which nonspecific activity replaces goal-directed actions.

Equally important, however, is that once such rhythmicities were expressed, infants opportunistically used them for specific intentional purposes. For example, I saw many examples of infants shaking and banging objects, kicking during interruptions of feeding or when mother appeared, or bouncing as a seemingly deliberate exploratory or play behavior (Thelen, 1981a). Here, infants performed what Piaget (1952) called *circular reactions*: repetitions of actions that produced interesting results. If the natural oscillations of the arms led to interesting noises from the grasped object, then infants appeared able to intentionally repeat those oscillations, presumably by creating the energetic conditions that allowed such oscillations to emerge. (I will give a more mechanistic explanation of this later in the chapter.) When, in turn, more focused skills such as fine manipulation developed, rhythmic exploration decreased.

The point is that we need not invoke any special purpose devices or dedicated developmental stages to explain these developmental phenomena. Infants act to meet goals; they perceive a situation and assemble whatever skills they possess to attain some need. Natural oscillations emerge when either the goal is not perceived or the means to attain it is not fully developed, and when intention does not match skill. Likewise, oscillations may substitute for more focused behavior when either the skill and its underlying neuromotor mechanisms are deficient, or the environment does not afford more functional actions. As I will suggest later, it may be these *processes* that link the normal stereotypies of infancy to those of nonnormal populations, rather than a straight developmental continuity.

Given this general framework, a number of more specific questions can be asked. What are the neuromotor and contextual mechanisms that produce these rhythmical movements? Why do they appear and disappear? What is the relation between oscillations and movements more specifically directed toward a goal? We can begin to answer these questions by detailed examination of particular infant stereotypies.

147

Infant Kicking: Mechanisms of Spontaneous Limb Oscillations

In this section, I will describe studies of one common infant rhythmical stereotypy—kicking of the legs. This behavior is common from the newborn period, is most frequent during 3 to 6 months of age, and declines as infants learn to crawl, stand, and walk. As with other stereotypies, kicking is seen in young infants mainly when they are excited or fussy, but later in the first year, kicking also appears to function as a communicative and exploratory activity.

The question to be addressed here is, why oscillation? What is the nature of the neuromotor organization that supports this class of oscillatory behaviors?

Our first studies documented the time and space patterning of leg kicks in young infants (Thelen, Bradshaw, & Ward, 1981; Thelen & Fisher, 1983b). Traditionally, movements in the first months of life have been described as random and uncoordinated. We found, in contrast, that leg kicks were indeed highly organized, rhythmic, and stereotyped at the kinematic level. Young infants kicked by simultaneously flexing and extending all three joints of one leg; hip, knee, and ankle moved together in often near perfect synchrony (Figure 6). The timing of the movement phases was similarly constrained, with the flexion phases taking about 300 ms and, whereas extensions were somewhat longer in duration, they were not randomly distributed (Figure 7). Likewise, infants showed some regularity of coordination between the legs. In the first months, they either kicked one leg alone or kicked in regular alternation (Thelen, 1985).

From the kinematic data alone, one might infer a number of neurological control models. The regularity of timing and coordination might be controlled by a detailed *central pattern generator,* as has been described for locomotor control in other species (Grillner, 1975). In this model, it would be assumed that the regularity was a function of the wiring in the brain or spinal cord, with specific excitatory and inhibitory connections that produced both the simultaneity of coordination within the limb, and the alternating coordination between limbs. Another model, equally plausible from kinematic data alone, might be a *reflex chain model.* Here the

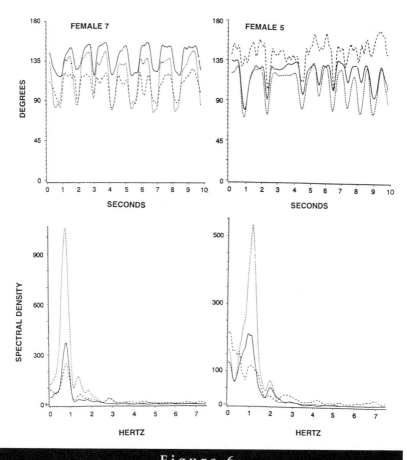

Figure 6

Joint angular rotations and spectral density plots of spontaneous kicking in two 4-week-old infants. In both plots, the solid line is the hip joint, the short-dashed line is the knee joint, and the long-dashed line is the ankle joint. Note the close synchrony of rotation of all three joints and the strong periodicity around 1 Hz. From *Journal of Motor Behavior, 15*, 353–377. Reprinted with permission of the Helen Dwight Reid Educational Foundation. Published by Heldref Publications, 1319 18th St., NW, Washington, DC, 20036-1802. © 1983.

rhythmicity would result from the sequential triggering of simple reflexes such as the withdrawal reflex, where the leg is rapidly flexed, and the cross-extensor reflex, where stimulation of one limb leads to flexion in the stimulated leg and extension in the opposite leg (Barnes, Crutchfield, Heriza, & Herdman, 1990).

Patterns of muscle activation revealed another picture, however (The-

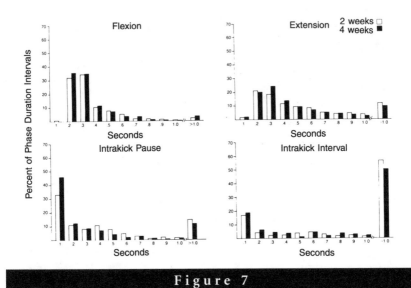

Figure 7

Frequency histograms of temporal durations of flexion and extension phases in spontaneous kicking in 2-week-old (clear bars) and 4-week-old (solid bars) infants. These are averaged data (n = 18 at 2 weeks; n = 19 at 4 weeks), 30 kicks per infant. Reprinted with permission of the Helen Dwight Reid Educational Foundation. Published by Heldref Publications, 1319 18th St., NW, Washington, DC, 20036-1802. © 1983.

len & Fisher, 1983b). Underlying this kinematic complexity—within limb coordination, timing invariances, interlimb coordination—were relatively simple patterns of muscle activation. Electromyography (EMG) of the major muscle groups of the leg showed that kicks were initiated by nearly simultaneous co-contraction of both agonist and antagonist muscle groups. Extension, in contrast, was associated with very little or no phasic muscle activity. Indeed, the spatial and temporal order of the movement could not be explained by the muscle patterns alone: The muscle contractions were simple co-contractions at flexion, yet the leg kinematics showed more complex and coordinated flexions and extensions.

Where did the time-and-space patterns come from? The discrepancy between the simple EMG and the more patterned kicks can only be understood in relation to the dynamic, self-organizing properties of the system. According to a dynamic view, movement form is not a product of central nervous system (CNS) commands alone, but arises as an emergent property of the neuromuscular anatomy; elastic properties of the muscles; and the energetic, intentional, and environmental context of the mover (Kugler, Kelso, & Turvey, 1980). As a dynamic system, the motor system behaves according to general principles governing nonlinear, complex systems. Such dynamic characterizations of human movement have been rigorously modeled and empirically confirmed (see Beek, 1989; Kugler & Turvey, 1987; Schöner & Kelso, 1988).

In particular, my colleagues and I have suggested that infant legs behave like mass-springs with a regular forcing function (energy kick; Thelen, Kelso, & Fogel, 1987). This was confirmed with studies at the level of joint torques. We used the techniques of *inverse dynamics* to understand the forces that actually move the limb joints when infants move (Schneider, Zernicke, Ulrich, Jensen, & Thelen, 1990). Typically, limbs are thought to move as a result of muscle contraction. But during natural movements, both gravity and inertial forces also contribute to the final pathway of the limb. The inertial forces result because any limb segment is mechanically linked to other moving segments. (Imagine vigorously shaking your arm at the shoulder while relaxing elbow and wrist.) By measuring accelerations of limb segments and estimating their masses, we used Newtonian equations of motion to calculate the forces from the active (muscle and tissue contraction) and passive (gravity and inertia) influences on the limbs. We found, in accordance with kinematic and EMG data, that in rhythmical kicking, while the flexion part of the cycle was initiated by active muscle contraction, the extension phase was passive, with gravity and inertial forces acting to pull the leg out and away from the body.

Thus, although the kicks had both temporal and spatial patterns, these patterns were not explicitly specified in the neural commands to the muscle. Rather, the patterns were emergent from both the energetic input to the legs in the form of muscle contraction, combined with the gravitational context, and the springy and inertial properties of the legs. The leg movements can be compared to those of a simple physical spring with a mass attached. When people impart energy to the spring, it oscillates with a regular period and amplitude that depends on the mass on the spring and its stiffness. As long as we periodically impart energy, the spring will, in a sense, "keep time" by its regular, rhythmic cycles, although there is no explicit clock in the spring itself or in the energy delivered to it.

Such a characterization of a rhythmical movement has important implications for understanding stereotyped behavior in general. The final form of the behavior must be a system property of the physical anatomy of the body segments involved, the neuromotor apparatus, the energetic status of the mover, and the particular support and gravitational context. Each of these contributes to the motor pattern, such that the pattern is a dynamic and emergent property. Although in some populations these patterns seem very stable, the stability may be as much a function of the body mechanics and the environment as a function of the neuromuscular control per se. Such a view also suggests that manipulations in these nonneural variables may act to destabilize the pattern, and indeed, it is well-known that environmental enrichment or distraction with alternative tasks disrupts pathological stereotypies. Thus, even behaviors that look "hard-wired" in the CNS may be amenable to intervention.

What Happens to Rhythmical Kicking?

By the last quarter of the first year, infants rarely perform bouts of rhythmical kicking. It is as important to understand the involution of this behavior as to understand its emergence. Indeed, it is precisely because these behaviors are dynamic and not hard-wired that infants soon move away from simple rhythmicities into more functionally diverse and adapted leg patterns.

First, it is important to note that even young infants can evidence some degree of control over their seemingly stereotyped movements. For example, Fisher and I used a ribbon attached to their ankles to allow 3-month-old infants to use their spontaneous kicks to move an overhead mobile (Thelen & Fisher, 1983a). In this circumstance, infants kicked more frequently and more vigorously to enjoy the motion and sound of the mobile. They were not intractably locked into a particular rhythm.

In addition, there are developmental changes in spontaneous kicking that reflect the lability of these patterns. The most dramatic is the increasing differentiation of the holistic pattern into more individually controlled segments. This differentiation was apparent both in coordination within the joints and between the patterns of two legs (Thelen, 1985). For instance, in young infants movements of the hip, knee, and ankle, considered pairwise, showed a high correlation; the joints flexed and extended in tight synchrony. However, by the middle of the first year, this tight coordination dissolved, and infants moved their joints more individually. Such individuation is necessary, of course, to free the system from rigid patterning to allow more flexible and adaptive patterns of coordination and control. Recently, we observed interjoint differentiation at the level of control of forces (Jensen, Ulrich, Thelen, Schneider, & Zernicke, 1995). Although early kicks were tightly coordinated, the infants were exerting most of the muscle force at the hip joint. The knee and ankle moved more as a passive consequence of the forces at the hip. Later in the first year, infants could control forces at both the hip and the knee.

ENTRAINMENT OF EARLY CYCLIC BEHAVIOR

It is most important to consider that although the transient rhythmicities of infancy may involute, the *potential* to produce cyclic behavior remains, albeit in more functional and environmentally entrained forms. (By *entrainment* I mean coupled to events or objects in the environment.) For example, evidence suggests that the capacity for rhythmic alternation of the legs in kicking is reasserted in various forms of later locomotion. The continuity became apparent in studies of treadmill-elicited stepping during infancy (Thelen, 1986; Thelen & Ulrich, 1991). In infants as young as 1 month of age, a small, motorized treadmill elicited coordinated, alternating steps. Step frequency and coordination continued to improve through age 6 or 7 months. What is remarkable about treadmill stepping, in addition to the mature-looking form of the within-limb coordination, is the precision and sensitivity of the between-limb phasing. For example, Thelen, Ulrich, and Niles (1987) found that infants maintained an alternating pattern even when one foot was driven on a belt moving at twice the speed of the belt supporting the opposite leg.

Infants use the same anatomical structures to step on the treadmill and to kick spontaneously. What differs, of course, is the context. The treadmill pulls the legs back and imparts a stretch to the muscles and tendons, which is detected by the infant. This signal from the stretched muscles acts as an entraining event, triggering the swing forward of one leg while inhibiting the swing forward of the opposite leg. Thus, although infants will often spontaneously kick in a cyclic and alternating pattern, the pattern becomes increasingly more stable when it is entrained to an environmental event, in this case, the moving treadmill. Presumably, the same capability to rhythmically alternate is later tapped by independent locomotion. There the entraining feedback is a consequence of the infants' own movements of forward propulsion, which similarly provide stretch of the standing leg.

The treadmill phenomenon supports the view of normal transient stereotypies as the natural oscillations of a dynamic system seen when infants have insufficient control to produce more environmentally appropriate matches between their goals and their actions. The treadmill manipulation shows that the system is indeed entrainable to environmental triggers, although in this case, independently of the intentional goals of the infant. In normal development, then, we can suggest that the same neural and energetic substrate that supports these transient rhythmicities also produces more goal-corrected actions. The task of the infant is not simply to inhibit the rhythmic movements, but to indeed appropriate and redirect this inherent organization to more task-appropriate ends.

A Dynamic Interpretation

In earlier work, I have characterized the movements of infants in dynamic terms as a series of attractors, which are the low-dimensional configurations in time and space of the preferred patterns of coordination (Thelen, 1989). Traditionally, attractors are depicted as trajectories on a *phase plane*, which plots the displacement of the movement versus its velocity. Phase planes are useful because they capture, as one function, the time–space behavior of the system and also, by inference, some characteristics of its energetic and control status. For example, consider a simple system—a spring with a mass attached. If one imparts energy to the spring, it will oscillate and eventually the oscillations will damp out and the spring will reach an equilibrium position. It will look like Figure 8A on the phase plane. In contrast, if one gives the spring a periodic energy pulse, it would continue to cycle, as in Figure 8B, and not show the damping to a single equilibrium position. In either case, the frequency and amplitude of the oscillations would depend on the stiffness of the spring and the mass attached.

The rhythmical movements of infants do indeed have the characteristics of cyclic attractors, and especially forced-mass springs, on the phase plane. Consider Figure 9, which plots the angular rotations of the knee joint versus the angular velocity of a series of kicks in a 2-week-old and 3-month-old infant. Notice in both examples how the trajectories of the successive cycles lie closely on top of each other, suggesting that the movement time–space characteristics are highly repeatable. Note also that these kicks (especially in the 2 week old) have similar topologies as the pendulums described in Figure 8A. The flattened top of the 3-month-old circles shows that while flexion was vigorous, extension in several kicks was slow (low and steady velocity). This suggests that between 2 weeks and 3 months, there may be a change of control strategy, with the additional ability to control and brake the leg appearing at the older age.

These exemplars, then, point out the more general developmental process, of the appropriation of the natural oscillation and the transformation into more environmentally sensitive movements. In this case, infants were kicking while held in an upright posture, where damping and braking a vigorous extension demonstrates a type of adaptive control. In fact, adults used a more controlled extension when asked to mimic infant kicks in this posture (Jensen et. al., 1995). The conversion of natural oscillations to voluntary actions is better demonstrated however, with movements of the upper limb, which I address in the next section.

Rhythmical Movements and Learning to Reach

An important class of rhythmical movements is associated with the transition to the first abilities to reach and grasp. In this section, I describe a

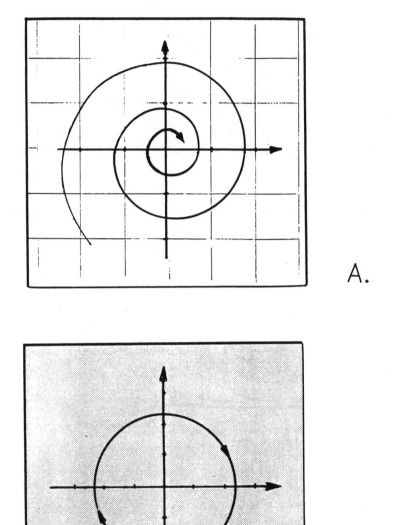

A.

B.

Figure 8

(A) Phase plane depiction of the motions of a damped mass spring. The phase plane plots the displacement of the movement versus its velocity. (B) Phase plane depiction of the motions of a forced spring.

recent study that detailed rhythmical flapping and rhythmical hand–mouth oscillations. In particular, I show the mechanisms by which oscillators (behaving like cyclic attractors) become converted by the infant into discrete movements.

The development of the skill of reaching has been the subject of numerous research studies (e.g., Fetters & Todd, 1987; Halverson, 1931; von Hofsten, 1979; Mathew & Cook, 1990; White, Castle, & Held, 1964). However, these studies have looked at changes in the actual reach movement itself, the directed arm extension toward the desired object. My colleagues and I have presented a different view of reaches as emerging from, and embedded in, an ongoing movement context (Thelen, Corbetta, & Spencer, in press). When viewed this way, it becomes evident that this ongoing movement context is often rhythmic and stereotyped in character. Thus, depending on the energy level of the infant, reaches may emerge from a more general oscillatory process.

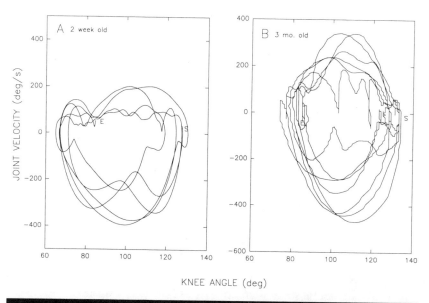

Figure 9

Phase plane depictions of repetitive kicking in a (A) 2-week-old and (B) 3-month-old infant. The angular rotations of the knee joint are plotted versus their velocities. S = start of movement, and E = end of movement.

The study involved 4 infants, who were observed weekly from 3 weeks until 30 weeks of age, and every other week thereafter until they were 1 year old. Infants were tested in a nearly upright infant seat, with a wide fabric band providing stabilizing postural support. We recorded movements in 14-second trials, during which we presented an attractive toy at midline 5 to 6 seconds after the trial began so that we captured not only the reach trajectory, but the movements preceding and following the reach itself. In this way, we captured the whole context of reaching.

First, we noted striking individual differences in how infants first learned to reach (Thelen et al., 1993). These differences were related foremost to the typical energy level of the infants. Two of the infants were especially active. They were energetic and forceful in all their movements, and they especially waved and flapped their arms. The other two infants were more quiet and showed much less overall body movement. The two active infants first reached by swiping at the toy and learning to damp down their excessive force and speed. In contrast, the two quiet infants had to impart sufficient muscle contraction to lift their arms against gravity and extend them up and out toward the toys. Their first reaches were slower and more coordinated.

Rhythmical oscillations were especially characteristic of the high-energy infants. In Figure 10, I present two examples of these infants' spontaneous movements, that is, their movements before they learned to actually reach and contact the toy. The examples, which are 14 seconds in length, are the movements of the hand, plotted to show the three-dimensional trajectory of the hand, the temporal characteristics of the hand movement, and the dynamics of the phase plane. On the phase plane, these movements have topological characteristics similar to the dynamics of a mass-spring that is being periodically forced and continues to oscillate although the distances and velocities of the movements vary.

How do these infants convert these oscillations into directed reaches? The problem can be stated dynamically as how they transform a periodic attractor to a point attractor, that is, into an attractor with a stable equilibrium point. Our evidence suggested that infants indeed used their muscle contractions effectively to damp down the spring-like qualities of the

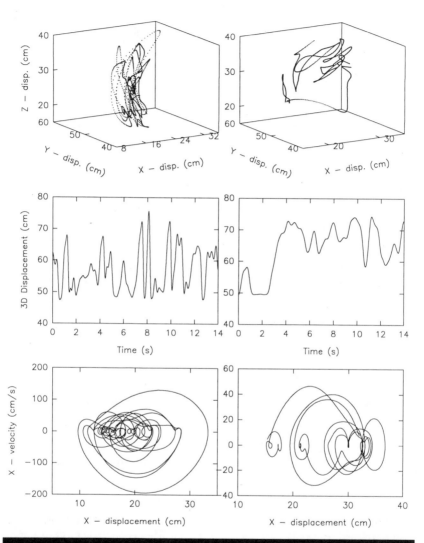

Figure 10

Various representations of the spontaneous arm movements of two infants before they could reach and grasp. The top panels show the 3-D trajectory of the hand movement. The x axis is the lateral (front-to-back), the y axis is the medial (across midline), and the z axis is up and down. Both infants are using their right hands; movements are directed across body to midline. The middle panels show the 3-displacement (resultant) of the hand as a time series, emphasizing the rhythmic nature of the movement. The bottom panels are the same movement plotted on the phase plane, but for only the displacement in the x (front-to-back) direction.

159

arms and, thus, reduce the tendency of the spring to oscillate (Thelen et al., 1993). Specifically, we believed that the infants changed the stiffness of the arm-spring system by muscle co-contraction in order to bring the hand to an equilibrium point, the location of the toy. In Figure 11, this process is illustrated on the phase plane by showing in two early reaches the actual conversion of cyclic movements to an equilibrium point. Figure 11A is a reach at the very first week of reaching. Note that the phase plane has the characteristics of spontaneous flapping movements seen in Figure 10, that is, high velocity, large amplitudes and a continuous, smooth amplitude–velocity relation. Essentially, this infant was using the flap to swipe at the toy. By the very next week (Figure 11B), the infant has learned to modulate these spring-like dynamics. Here, although he starts the reach with a large, fast movement, he slows down before the final approach to the toy, indicated by the flattened, slow velocity values. Indeed, the reach is carved from the very same oscillatory dynamics as the flapping movements.

These data illustrate two points: first, as I hypothesized previously, that transient rhythmical stereotypies are expressions of the natural oscillatory properties of the neuromotor system before good voluntary control under particular energetic constraints. Second, these data show that the same dynamics that underlie these nongoal-corrected movements are used for more adaptive and intentional actions. That is, the infants appeared to use the same spring-like qualities to move into the reach itself. Although not all infants reached by first flapping, this is powerful evidence that the potential for rhythmicity is inherent in the system itself.

Finally, I would like to introduce a rhythmical stereotypy discovered in this longitudinal reaching data and described by Smith (1992). When infants reach and grab objects, they very frequently transport them to their mouths. In tracing the developmental course of hand-to-mouth and object-to-mouth behavior, Smith found that just before infants were able to grasp objects effectively, they showed a highly stereotyped bimanual cyclic behavior of reaching out toward the object, grasping both hands together, and transporting the clasped hands to the mouth. As in other stereotypies, this behavior is transient—it appears just before successful arm-

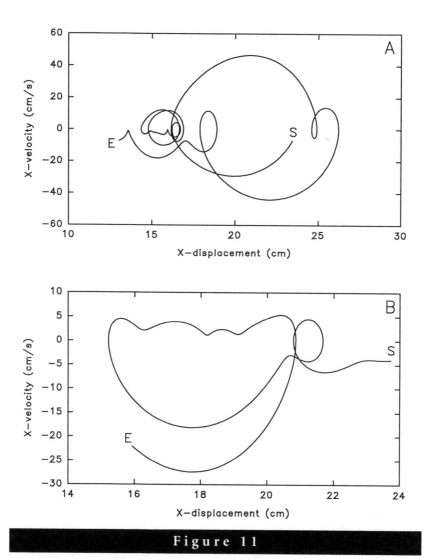

Figure 11

Reaches in one infant at 15 weeks (week of first reaching) and 16 weeks as depicted on the phase plane. S = start of segment; E = contact with toy. (A) Reaching movement is a high-velocity swipe, continuous with the flap, depicted as the large, rounded upper loop. (B) Infant starts with a high-velocity movement, but slows down before contacting the toy, seen as the flattened loop on the phase plane.

extended reaching and within a week or two, when infants can grab toys, becomes less repetitive and disappears, although bringing the object to the mouth persists for many months. On the phase plane, the movements look as in Figure 11, which captures the continuous loop of cyclic repetitions toward the toy location and then to the mouth. Also as before, infants must gain control of the movement in relation to the environment—in this case, actually grabbing the toy—but both the stereotyped and goal-corrected movement rely on the same dynamic substrate.

CONCLUSION

Our developmental data provide strong evidence that rhythmicity is not a simple product of a central rhythm generator that becomes variously inhibited or released. Rather, oscillation appears to be a natural state of human neuromotor systems under specific constraints, which include tonus, energetic status, and the degree of voluntary control over the limbs. Such systems can display dynamic characteristics of oscillating physical systems. In particular, infant arms and legs can behave like mass springs. Recently Goldfield (1993; Goldfield, Kay, & Warren, 1993) has made a similar claim for two whole-body stereotypies, rocking on hands and knees and bouncing in a Jolly Jump-up. In all cases, infants must effectively "tune" the springs to match their intentional goals—bounce, move forward, or bring the hands to the toy or toy to the mouth. Thus, one may say that the voluntary behavior is carved out of this potentially oscillating dynamic.

It seems reasonable to assume that both central and peripheral pathologies can also induce stereotyped behavior by interrupting voluntary control at any number of levels. If sensory deprivation removes the goal or task, the system may well "free-run" and oscillate but, in turn, these oscillations are maintained because they then provide needed stimulation. That is, the oscillation may replace more adaptive behavior as a preferred attractor or motor habit. Likewise, lesions and drugs may interrupt normal control pathways, again releasing this natural spring-like behavior. Disturbances of limb compliance control, as in Parkinsonian disease, may also allow the natural resonant frequencies of the system to be displayed.

The message from the normal infant data is that in some cases, providing appropriate environmental support may redirect the system out of the repetitive habit and into more adaptive actions.

REFERENCES

Barnes, M. L., Crutchfield, C., Heriza, C. B., & Herdman, S. (1990). *Reflex and vestibular aspects of motor control, motor development, and motor learning.* Atlanta, GA: Stokesville.

Beek, P. J. (1989). *Juggling dynamics.* Amsterdam: Free University Press.

Berkson, G. (1967). Abnormal stereotyped motor acts. In J. Zubin & H. Hunt (Eds.), *Comparative psychopathology: Animal and human* (pp. 76–94). New York: Grune & Stratton.

Fetters, L., & Todd, J. (1987). Quantitative assessment of infant reaching movements. *Journal of Motor Behavior, 19,* 147–166.

Goldfield, E. C. (1993). Dynamical systems in development: Action systems. In L. B. Smith & E. Thelen (Eds.), *Dynamic approaches to development: Applications.* Cambridge, MA: MIT Press.

Goldfield, E. C., Kay, B. A., & Warren, W. H., Jr. (1993). Infant bouncing: The assembly and tuning of action systems. *Child Development, 64,* 1128–1142.

Grillner, S. (1975). Locomotion in vertebrates: Central mechanisms and reflex interaction. *Physiological Reviews, 55,* 247–304.

Halverson, H. M. (1931). An experimental study of prehension in infants by means of systematic cinema records. *Genetic Psychology Monographs, 10,* 107–286.

Hofsten, C., von (1979). Development of visually directed reaching: The approach phase. *Journal of Human Movement Studies, 5,* 160–178.

Hutt, C., & Hutt, J. S. (1965). Effect of environmental complexity upon stereotyped behaviours in children. *Animal Behaviour, 13,* 1–4.

Jensen, J. L., Ulrich, B. D., Thelen, E., Schneider, K., & Zernicke, R. F. (1995). Adaptive dynamics of the leg movement patterns of human infants: Age-related changes in kicks. *Journal of Motor Behavior, 27,* 366–374.

Kaufman, M. E., & Levitt, H. (1965). A study of three stereotyped behaviors in institutionalized mental defectives. *American Journal of Mental Deficiency, 69,* 467–473.

Kravitz, H., & Boehm, J. (1971). Rhythmic habit patterns in infancy: Their sequences, age of onset, and frequency. *Child Development, 42,* 399–413.

Kugler, P. N., Kelso, J. A. S., & Turvey, M. T. (1980). On the concept of coordinative structures as dissipative structures: I. Theoretical lines of convergence. In G. E. Stelmach & J. Requin (Eds.), *Tutorials in motor behavior* (pp. 3–47). New York: North Holland.

Kugler, P. N., & Turvey, M. T. (1987). *Information, natural law, and the self-assembly of rhythmic movement.* Hillsdale, NJ: Erlbaum.

Lourie, R. S. (1949). The role of rhythmic patterns in childhood. *American Journal of Psychiatry, 105,* 653–660.

MacLean, W. E., Ellis, D. N., Galbreath, H. N., Halpern, L. F., & Baumeister, A. A. (1991). Rhythmic motor behavior of preambulatory motor impaired, Down syndrome, and nondisabled children: A comparative analysis. *Journal of Abnormal Child Psychology, 19,* 319–330.

Mathew, A., & Cook, M. (1990). The control of reaching movements by young infants. *Child Development, 61,* 1238–1258.

Piaget, J. (1952). *The origins of intelligence in children.* New York: International Universities Press.

Schneider, K., Zernicke, R. F., Ulrich, B. D., Jensen, J. L., & Thelen, E. (1990). Understanding movement control in infants through the analysis of limb intersegmental dynamics. *Journal of Motor Behavior, 22,* 493–520.

Schöner, G., & Kelso, J. A. S. (1988). Dynamic pattern generation in behavioral and neural systems. *Science, 239,* 1513–1520.

Smith, G. A. (1992, May). *Hand-to-mouth behaviors in 5- to 30-week old infants.* Paper presented at the Eighth International Conference on Infant Studies, Miami Beach, FL.

Thelen, E. (1979). Rhythmical stereotypies in normal human infants. *Animal Behaviour, 27,* 699–715.

Thelen, E. (1981a). Kicking, rocking, and waving: Contextual analysis of rhythmical stereotypies in normal human infants. *Animal Behaviour, 29,* 3–11.

Thelen, E. (1981b). Rhythmical behavior in infancy: An ethological perspective. *Developmental Psychology, 17,* 237–257.

Thelen, E. (1985). Developmental origins of motor coordination: Leg movements in human infants. *Developmental Psychobiology, 18,* 1–22.

Thelen, E. (1986). Treadmill-elicited stepping in seven-month-old infants. *Child Development, 57,* 1498–1506.

Thelen, E. (1989). Self-organization in developmental processes: Can systems approaches work? In M. Gunnar & E. Thelen (Eds.), *Systems in development: The*

Minnesota Symposia in Child Psychology (Vol. 22, pp. 77–117). Hillsdale, NJ: Erlbaum.

Thelen, E., Bradshaw, G., & Ward, J. A. (1981). Spontaneous kicking in month-old infants: Manifestations of a human central locomotor program. *Behavioral and Neural Biology, 32,* 45–53.

Thelen, E., Corbetta, D., Kamm, K., Spencer, J. P., Schneider, K., & Zernicke, R. F. (1993). The transition to reaching: Mapping intention and intrinsic dynamics. *Child Development, 64,* 1058–1098.

Thelen, E., Corbetta, D., & Spencer, J. P. (in press). The development of reaching during the first year: The role of movement speed. *Journal of Experimental Psychology: Human Perception and Performance.*

Thelen, E., & Fisher, D. M. (1983a). From spontaneous to instrumental behavior: Kinematic analysis of movement changes during very early learning. *Child Development, 54,* 129–140.

Thelen, E., & Fisher, D. M. (1983b). The organization of spontaneous leg movements in newborn infants. *Journal of Motor Behavior, 15,* 353–377.

Thelen, E., Kelso, J. A. S., & Fogel, A. (1987). Self-organizing systems and infant motor development. *Developmental Review, 7,* 39–65.

Thelen, E., & Ulrich, B. D. (1991). Hidden skills: A dynamic systems analysis of treadmill stepping during the first year. *Monographs of the Society for Research in Child Development, 58* (1, Serial No. 223).

Thelen, E., Ulrich, B., & Niles, D. (1987). Bilateral coordination in human infants: Stepping on a split-belt treadmill. *Journal of Experimental Psychology: Human Perception and Performance, 13,* 405–410.

White, B. L., Castle, P., & Held, R. (1964). Observations on the development of visually-directed reaching. *Child Development, 35,* 349–364.

Wolff, P. H. (1968). Stereotypic behavior and development. *Canadian Psychologist, 9,* 474–483.

8

Dimensions of Disintegration in the Stereotyped Locomotion Characteristic of Parkinsonism and Autism

Philip Teitelbaum, Ralph G. Maurer, Joshua Fryman,
Osnat B. Teitelbaum, Joel Vilensky, and
Margaret P. Creedon

The term *stereotypies* is usually applied to repetitive, seemingly purposeless, or even maladaptive movements of part of the body. It has also been applied to movements of the whole body in a circumscribed area, as in a cage, where the focus is on the repetition and seeming aimlessness of the behavior. Stereotypy is not generally used to describe unconstrained locomotion in an open field, which is the subject of this chapter. However, such locomotion may indeed be extremely stereotyped, as revealed in some animal models (Cheng, Schallert, DeRyck, & Teitelbaum, 1981; Chesire & Teitelbaum, 1982; Golani, Wolgin, & Teitelbaum, 1979; Levitt & Teitelbaum, 1975; Pellis, Pellis, Chesire, Rowland, & Teitelbaum, 1987; Schallert, DeRyck, & Teitelbaum, 1980; Schallert, Whishaw, Ramirez,

We thank Iris Klein, the director of Sav-Yom, the Daycare Center for the Elderly at Emek Yizrael Regional Council, and the very able members of her staff for helping P. T. to observe and to videotape some of the phenomena of Parkinson's disease described here. We thank the staff of the library of the high school at Kibbutz Misra in Israel, who served as a control group in our videos of gait. We also thank the members of Kibbutz Merhavia for their hospitality, and for providing computer facilities that enabled P. T. to work on this chapter. In particular, we wish to thank the people suffering from Parkinson's disease who graciously allowed us to film their gait under sometimes taxing conditions so that others might learn. Finally, we owe special thanks to Shar Yashuv Uri of Kibbutz Beit Ha Shita, who explained to us the ingenious methods he had worked out to help improve his own parkinsonian gait. His techniques form the basis of several of the principles we have formulated here.

& Teitelbaum, 1978; Szechtman, Eilam, Teitelbaum, & Golani, 1988; Szechtman, Ornstein, Teitelbaum, & Golani, 1985; Teitelbaum, Pellis, & DeVietti, 1990). For instance, at a certain stage during its recovery from the akinesia produced by large bilateral electrolytic lesions in the lateral hypothalamus in an animal model of parkinsonism (see Teitelbaum, 1986), the brain-damaged animal seems to be exploring the open field as though it were hungry because it stops to nibble at food that it encounters during the course of its locomotion. However, if it wanders into a corner, the animal may become trapped for long periods, engaging in a stereotyped, repetitive sequence of head-scanning reactions to the walls and floor of the enclosure (Levitt & Teitelbaum, 1975). It is not the partial enclosure that physically traps the animal. What does so is the limited number of behavioral reactions that the damaged brain can provide in such a configuration of surfaces. Such a *behavioral trap* (Schallert et al., 1980) shatters the "perceptual illusion of adaptive wholeness" ordinarily created by locomotion from place to place (Teitelbaum et al., 1990, p. 170). It reveals that even in an open field, during several stages of partial reintegration after brain damage, locomotion can be an extremely disintegrated, simplified form (Golani et al., 1979).

It seems to us, therefore, that a more general definition of stereotypy should be adopted. That is, a stereotypy is a disintegrated form of behavior that can, under appropriate circumstances, be highly repetitive and seemingly purposeless. It can be induced by drugs or brain damage in an adult, or even be due to incomplete normal development. This way of looking at it allows us to understand the nature of a stereotypy more fully by emphasizing that one should explore the dimensions and degree of disintegration relative to the normal fully integrated adult, by specifying which subcomponents remain operative and which do not, and by showing which environmental or self-generated stimuli operate on those subcomponents to produce the particular form of stereotypy that is being displayed. The understanding of the hierarchical level of remaining function that this approach provides promotes the application not only of drug treatment as replacement therapy for tissue that has been rendered inoperative, but also of a combination of drugs and behavioral therapy for the

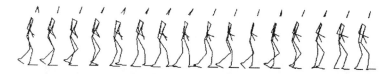

Figure 1

Stick-figure resynthesis of the gait of a child with autism, using the PEAK 2D motion analysis system. Note that unlike the normal gait, the arms are held flexed in front of the body and do not swing back and forth as the legs step.

released undamaged systems that remain functional but imbalanced. It follows also that one may learn about stereotyped behavior by studying disintegrated forms of locomotion.

We extended this line of thought by studying disintegrated locomotion in people. For instance, in some respects, the gait of children with autism has been found to parallel that of adults suffering from Parkinson's disease (Damasio & Maurer, 1978; Vilensky, Damasio, & Maurer, 1981). In these early works, only the quantitative aspects of the movement of the legs were measured. Compared to normal children, children with autism take shorter, slower steps.

When we reviewed the films of Vilensky et al. (1981), it was clear that some children with autism do not swing their arms as they walk. This similarity to parkinsonism had been reported by Vilensky et al. (1981). Lack of associated arm movement during walking in early infantile autism has also been reported by Segawa and Nomura (1991). Our stick-figure resyntheses[1] confirmed these earlier observations (see Figure 1).

In addition, we noticed that the arms of some of the children with autism, though they did not alternate during walking and were held in front of the body like that of many adults with parkinsonism, appeared to be more elevated (compare Figure 1 with Figure 2A). We hypothesized that this might be a compensatory balancing reaction in response to postural instability. Indeed, one of the present authors had earlier observed

---

[1]For stick-figure resynthesis, we used the PEAK 2D Video/Computer Motion Measurement System that was supplied by PEAK Performance Technologies, Inc., 7388 S. Revere Parkway, Suite 601, Englewood, Colorado 80112.

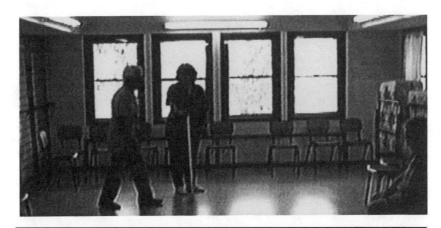

Figure 2A

A person with Parkinson's disease walking naturally. His arms swing very little, and he walks slowly, with relatively short steps.

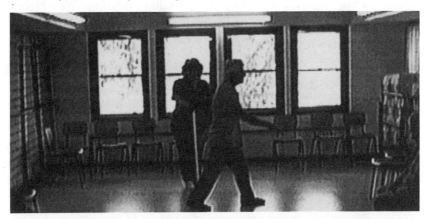

Figure 2B

When asked to swing his arms while walking, he immediately walks faster, takes longer steps, and holds head more erect.

postural instability in children with autism, which also was documented in evaluations by occupational therapists (Creedon, 1991).

While seated, some people with Parkinson's disease do not raise their arms to maintain their balance when they are tilted suddenly (Martin,

1967). Again, some children with autism also respond the same way (Creedon, 1992). We used Sydenham's method of template-matching (Faber, 1919/1978), which can be applied reiteratively to such parallels, as an heuristic guide to a more detailed descriptive analysis of each disorder. Thus, the similarities and possible differences between balancing reactions in parkinsonism versus those in autism suggested the need for specific additional comparisons of gait and of balancing reactions in each syndrome. Also, there is evidence that under certain circumstances people with Parkinson's disease cannot do two things at the same time (Caligiuri, Heindel, & Lohr, 1992). We wondered whether this might mean that they would not be able to continue to walk while concentrating on something else. The present chapter is a report of preliminary new observations on adults with Parkinson's disease and a review of earlier films of the gait of children with autism that are relevant to the questions mentioned.

METHODS

Some of the 16 mm-movie films of Vilensky et al. (1981), which documented leg movements during walking of normal versus autistic children, were converted to VHS $^1/_2$-inch videotape. We then applied Eshkol-Wachman Movement Notation (EWMN) to the analysis of the walking patterns.

Sav-Yom is a day-care center for the elderly in Israel that provides cultural, occupational, and physical therapy. Among the clients is a group of people with Parkinson's disease. After obtaining informed consent from eight people with Parkinson's disease, we videotaped their gait and the gait of an additional person with Parkinson's disease at Kibbutz Merhavia, as well as that of five normal elderly people (members of the staff of the library of the nearby high school at Kibbutz Misra). All videotaping was done by means of a hand-held Sony Hi-8 Camcorder. The mean age of the parkinsonian group was 70.2 years, ranging from 60 to 79. The mean age of the normal control group was 69.6 years, ranging from 57 to 80.

All of the numerical data about the size and speed of step reported in the present chapter were based on measurements taken directly frame-by-frame by hand from the image on the TV monitor. A rod of known length (either 1 m or 1.5 m) was held briefly by each subject at the beginning of each videotaped sequence so that absolute measurements of distances moved were always available. We also applied EWMN in frame-by-frame analysis to selected portions of the video material, in order to obtain greater understanding of the kinematics of the phenomena (Eshkol, 1980; Eshkol & Wachman, 1958).

The gait of all of the subjects was videotaped under the following conditions and in the same order:

1. The subject was asked to walk across the room, a distance of about 4 meters, and to turn around and walk back to the starting point. This was the baseline for comparison with the conditions that followed.
2. The subject was asked to walk the same course and deliberately swing his or her arms while walking.
3. The subject was asked to walk directly toward the camera, a distance of approximately 5 meters, and then to turn around and walk back to the starting point. This was the baseline for comparison with the next maneuver.
4. The subject was asked to walk the same course as in condition 3, this time heel-to-toe.
5. The subject was asked to walk the same course as in condition 4, again heel-to-toe, toward and away from the camera, this time raising both arms straight out to the side at shoulder level, like a person in the circus balancing while walking on a tightrope.
6. The subject was asked to walk back and forth across the field of view of the camera, as in condition 1.
7. The subject was asked to walk back and forth as in condition 6, but this time to say out loud some information available in rote memory (e.g., the alphabet in Hebrew) as he or she walked.
8. Finally, the subject was again asked to walk back and forth as in condition 6, but this time to count out loud backward by sevens from 100.

RESULTS AND DISCUSSION

The subjects with Parkinson's disease differed greatly in their degree of disintegration in locomotion and postural stability, even though all were being maintained by drug therapy. Only two out of nine subjects, S. Y. U. and S. A., were able to participate in all of the conditions.

Condition 1: When asked to walk back and forth across the room, S. Y. U. held his arms slightly bent, close to the front surface of his body, so that his hands were at about the level of the hips (see Figure 2A). In people with Parkinson's disease, this is a typical position of the arms during walking. Because S. Y. U. appeared to be more lightly affected than many parkinsonian patients, his arms did swing a little; however, they never swung behind his body as he walked, which is the normal character of arm swinging. In addition, he walked with a shuffling gait, putting more weight on his right leg, leaning forward and to the right, without the maintenance of midline symmetry.

Condition 2: When asked to walk as in condition 1, but deliberately swinging his arms, S. Y. U. did so. At first he moved each arm forward along with the leg on the opposite side, as is normal when the arms swing automatically. After he had finished the traverse and had stopped to turn around, he resumed walking, but this time he swung each arm forward along with the ipsilateral leg. (Note that in the normal person, this ordinarily happens only when one consciously thinks about it, not when arm movement automatically accompanies the gait.) Such ipsilaterally synchronous arm–leg movement caused the steps to be bigger (an average of 1.45 ft per step without arm swinging vs. 1.86 ft per step while swinging the arms ipsilaterally, an increase of 28%) and faster (2.24 ft per second without arm swinging vs. 3.56 ft per second while swinging the arms, an increase of 59%). The arm movement preceded each step, as though the subject with Parkinson's disease was giving a command with his arm to initiate the walking.

When such erroneous pairing of the arm and the leg on the same side occurred, the subject was asked to swing the opposite arm forward along with the leg that moved forward. As with ipsilateral arm swing, the effect was also quite marked—S. Y. U.'s posture was more erect and his steps were longer and faster (about as fast as with ipsilateral arm swinging: ipsilateral 3.56 ft per second vs. 3.30 ft per second when the arm contralateral to the forward-stepping leg swung forward). When walking without swinging his arms, the size of a representative step was 24 cm. (A step is the distance from the toes of the rear foot before leaving the ground to the heel of the front foot while on the ground.) When walking while swinging his arms contralaterally to each leg, the subject's step measured 44 cm—an increase of 83% (Figures 2A and 2B). The change in step size was also obvious in the videotape: 9 steps without arm swing versus 6 steps to cross the same distance while swinging the arms. Clearly, consciously swinging his arms improved the subject's gait as he walked.

Similar results were obtained with S. A. He walked faster (2.87 ft per second without swinging his arms and 3.38 ft per second while swinging them, an increase of 18%) and took larger steps (1.42 ft per step without arm swing and 1.66 ft per step while swinging his arms, an increase of 17%).

These results also have been verified and extended in 10 subjects with Parkinson's disease in experiments subsequently carried out by our group at the University of Florida (Behrman et al., 1994).

Indirect augmentation via allied reflexes operates in people with Parkinson's disease to improve their gait. Reflexes that are allied with arm-swinging (which control step size and step rhythm) can act automatically to improve gait, but they are not brought into play when people with Parkinson's disease consciously direct themselves to walk forward because, for reasons still unknown, they do not spontaneously swing their arms when they walk.

While swinging his arms, S. Y. U. did walk with larger, faster steps in a way that suggested that he was more sure of himself. However, his shift of weight still differed from that of the normal person; he first tilted his weight forward and then stepped. (The fact that forward-body tilt precedes parkinsonian stepping [without swinging the arms] has been reported by Forrsberg, Johnels, & Steg, 1984.) This suggests that indirect augmentation via reflexes allied with walking is selective, not directly affecting those reflexes responsible for maintaining balance during the shift of weight in locomotion.

It should be noted that the marked improvement in gait induced by deliberately swinging the arms may be clearest and most marked only in the early stages of Parkinson's disease,[2] as in the case of S. Y. U., who was much less impaired in arm swing than the other patients in the group.

The fact that arm synchrony is quite labile in people with Parkinson's disease is highlighted by I. S., the third patient who participated in condition 2. As is shown in Figure 3 (A–E), his form of arm swing at first seemed quite bizarre and almost totally unsynchronized with his steps. His arms swung exaggeratedly up and down and reached a height in front of the body that is level with or above the shoulders, the way Russian soldiers march on parade. However, they swung up and down and crossed alongside each other in front of his body at an angle of about 45 degrees downward from the horizontal (see Figure 3D) rather than crossing in the vertical downward position as is normal. Also, the crossing point of the arms bore no relation in time to when the legs crossed alongside each other, though in the normal person arms and legs arrive at this neutral point simultaneously. Correspondingly, the participant's gait was not improved by swinging his arms as he walked. Indeed, it was worsened: he walked 22% more slowly.

In summary, in Figure 3, (a) the arms swing without maintaining the normal contralateral pattern; (b) the neutral point of the arms is shifted forward unrelated to the neutral point of the legs; (c) the body is tilted backward to counteract the forward position of the arms; (d) the body's shift of weight is decoupled from the stepping movements, occurring only after ground-support exists for both legs simultaneously; and (e) the vestibular control over the upper body, which enables it to remain vertical no matter what the arms and legs are doing, does not control the upper body, so that it is aligned with the legs rather than with gravity. This

---

[2]We thank Dr. Kenneth Heilman of the Neurology Department of the University of Florida for pointing out to us that we were able to see these phenomena in S. Y. U. because his was a mild degree of Parkinson's disease.

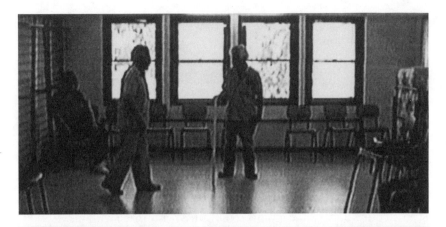

Figure 3A

Man with Parkinson's disease walking as usual without swinging his arms. Note his slightly forward-leaning erect posture and relatively short steps.

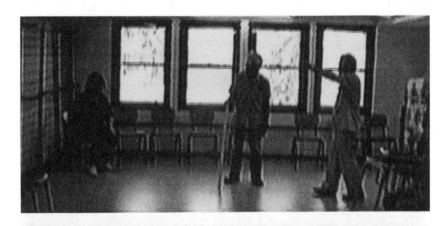

Figure 3B

When asked to swing his arms while walking, he begins by sweeping the left arm upward contralateral to the forward right step. Note the exaggerated upward swing of the left arm and the fact that the right arm does not swing behind the body. To compensate for the forward weight of the left arm, the body is tilted backward, causing the toes of the right foot to be lifted up. As in Figure 3E, the upward "reaching" of the left arm appears to trigger allied reflexes that indirectly help the ipsilateral leg to unweight and step forward.

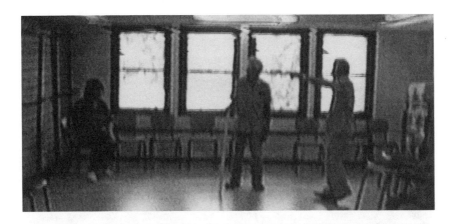

Figure 3 C

He swings his left leg forward almost to its neutral position, but the arm barely begins to descend.

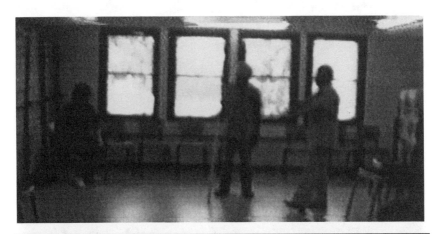

Figure 3 D

The arms reach a neutral point (aligned parallel to each other) about 45 degrees upward from the normal neutral point (parallel, vertically downward). The right heel does not release contact with the ground before contact is made with the left heel, indicating that shift of body weight does not occur until support by the ground is present in both legs.

(*Figure continues on next page.*)

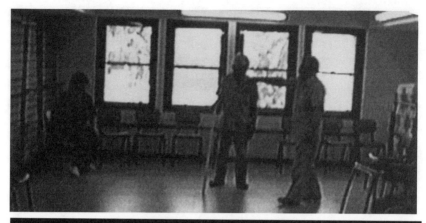

Figure 3E

The right arm's upward movement ends and the arm begins to "reach" forward, indirectly triggering allied reflexes that help the right leg to unweight and step forward.

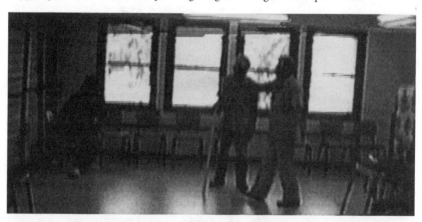

Figure 3F

The right arm remains up and reaches forward as the right leg steps forward and aligns ipsilaterally with the arm.

results in a severe inability to maintain anterior–posterior postural stability when swinging the arms while walking.

The form of arm swing displayed by I. S. fits some definitions of what constitutes a stereotypy; it is a repetitive action of parts of the body that seems maladaptive in the sense that it slows down the subject's speed of walking. Is it really maladaptive? A more detailed frame-by-frame analysis (using EWMN) of what happens during this seemingly bizarre form of arm swinging revealed that the arm swing of I. S. is actually a highly adaptive complex response to a conflict between the need to maintain stable equilibrium and the need to obey the instruction to swing the arms while walking.

Note first in Figure 3A (the man on the left) that when the participant walked as usual, without swinging his arms, he walked in an erect slightly forward-leaning posture. In Figure 3B (the man on the right), however, it is evident that as soon as he began to swing his left arm forward in a voluntary arm swing, he leaned his body backward as though compensating for a tendency to fall forward induced by the weight of the arm as it swung out in front of his body. As shown in Figures 3B and 3C, the backward-leaning was so great that the feet did not roll forward from heel contact onto the toes as he stepped forward. (Note that the toes of his right foot are elevated [Figure 3B and Figure 4] even as the left leg swings forward [Figure 3C].) So a new, complex, barely stable, anterior–posterior equilibrium was set up in response to the instruction to swing the arms; the arms swung, only in front of the participant's body, balancing and balanced by the now backward-leaning body and the neutral crossing point was displaced 45 degrees upward from the normal vertical-downward neutral point (see Figure 3D). In this backward-leaning position it is very difficult to unweight the leg that must be lifted from behind the body and swung forward. For instance, to aid the step of the left leg (see Figures 3B and 3C), the left arm swung upward exaggeratedly almost 45 degrees above shoulder level. This form of "reaching" upward indirectly triggered the allied postural reflexes of unweighting the leg on the same side, allowing the participant to step forward with it (Teitelbaum, Pellis, & Pellis, 1991). When the right leg had to step forward (Figure 3E), the normal contralateral synchrony of arm and leg was sacrificed in the interest of unweighting that leg while maintaining postural equilibrium at the same time. This man solved the problem—seemingly quite unconsciously—by keeping the ipsilateral (right) arm up at shoulder level and reaching forward slightly with it. This brought along the allied reflexes that facilitate the unweighting of the ipsilateral leg, allowing him to continue to walk, even though the normal contralateral synchrony was dispensed with (Figure 3).

Furthermore, written notation combined with frame-by-frame analysis revealed a decoupling between the participant's stepping movements and his shift of body weight (see Figures 4 and 5). Shift of weight is normally coupled with the step as it moves forward past the neutral point where both legs are side by side (frames 17, 50, 80, 108, etc. in Figure 4). In this man with parkinsonism, there was no shift of weight as the leg swung forward. Therefore, each leg reached its full forward position up in the air instead of contacting the ground at this point. So the leg had to be lowered back down to the ground from its fully extended position in the air in a kind of little "goosestep" (see frame 28 in Figure 5). Thus, in each step, only when stable equilibrium was achieved with support (ground

Figure 4 (facing page)

Sequence of 9 steps in a parkinsonian patient who is voluntarily swinging his arms while walking. (a) *Bar-lines:* A blackened, thicker, vertical line is a bar-line. Bar-lines denote the start or end of a movement. By looking at the bar-lines on the manuscript page, the relationship of legs to arms and of one leg to the other emerges clearly. One can see, for instance, that the arms start moving only toward the end of step 2 and change direction in the middle of step 3; that is, they are not synchronized with the steps. In step 2, it is apparent that the right leg starts moving only after the left has finished, whereas in step 7, the left leg starts moving while the right leg is still moving. (b) *Frame no.:* The video frame rate is 30 frames per second. The number in the frame space denotes the frame in which a movement starts or ends. If a movement starts on frame 1 and ends on frame 6, it lasted 6 frames. (c) *Roman numerals under each step:* These indicate the step number in the sequence. (d) *Signs:* S: A step. All steps are forward steps ((O)S). T: Touch (contact) of the feet with the ground. = : Release of contact with the ground. $\frac{(4)}{T}$: All of the foot except for the toes is in contact with the ground. $\frac{3}{4}$: Release of contact of the heel with the ground. $\frac{(4)}{T}$: Contact of the heel with the ground. ⋆: Appears only in the right arm space and means that the right arm position or movement was not visible, so we had to guess. [o] Neutral position. Both legs are alongside each other. [ô]: Crossing point ("neutral position") of the arms is 45 degrees in front of the body. ↓↑: When this appears in the arm spaces, it means (↑) upward, or (↓) downward movement. The arms are moving in the forward plane (0) throughout.

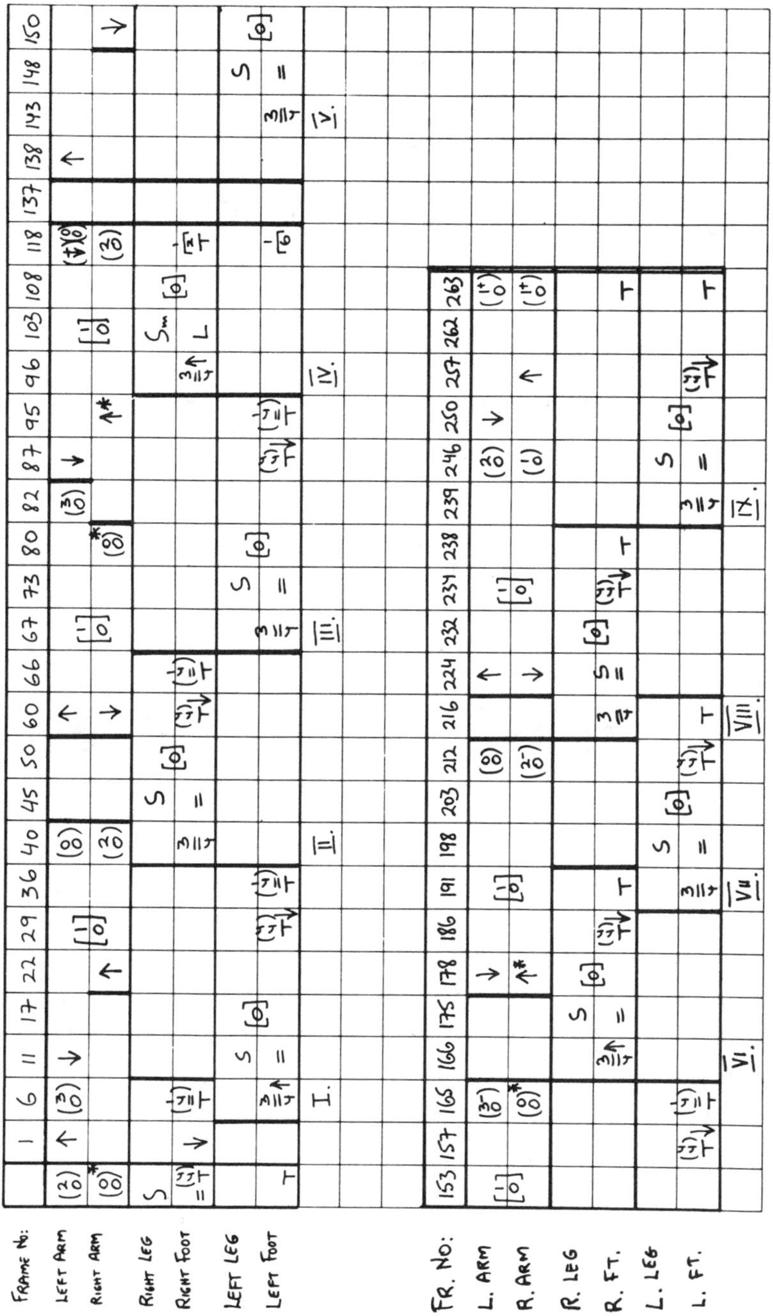
FRAME No:
LEFT ARM
RIGHT ARM
RIGHT LEG
RIGHT FOOT
LEFT LEG
LEFT FOOT
1 6 11 17 22 29 36 40 45 50 60 66 67 73 80 82 87 95 96 103 108 118 137 138 143 148 150
I. II. III. IV. V.
FR. NO:
L. ARM
R. ARM
R. LEG
R. FT.
L. LEG
L. FT.
153 157 165 166 175 178 186 191 198 203 212 216 224 232 234 238 239 246 250 257 262 263
VI. VII. VIII. IX.

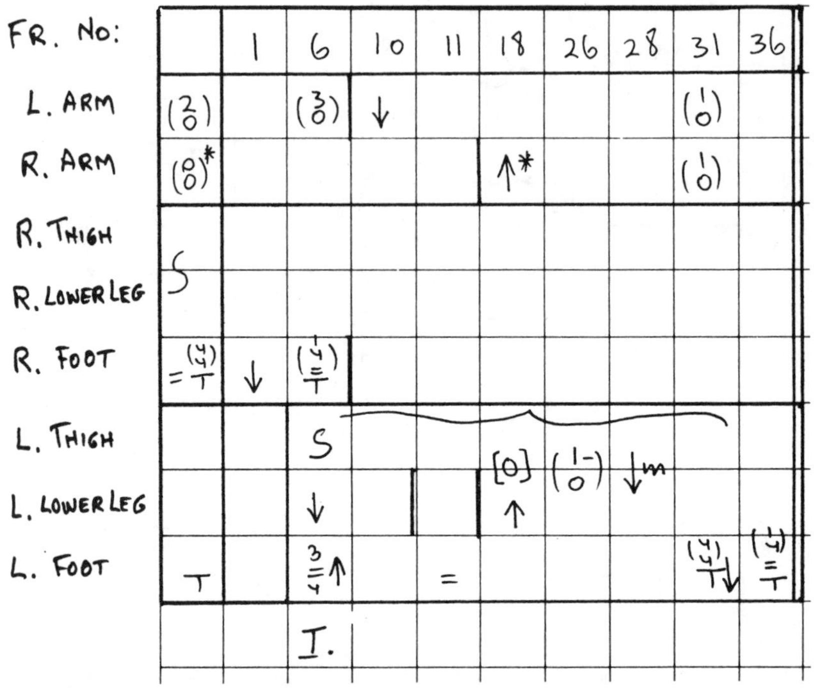

Figure 5

This is a more detailed notation of step 1 from Figure 4. (See Figure 4 note for meaning of symbols.) It highlights the decoupling of the shift of weight from the step movement. Note the sequence of the left leg in frames 18 through 28.

contact) by both legs at the same time did shift of body weight occur. Note that in each step the heel of the rear leg did not release contact with the ground until the forward swinging leg had established contact so that simultaneous support exists in both legs while the weight is being shifted. This is quite abnormal. Is it possible that in this man with parkinsonism a regression has occurred from the normal adult form of dynamic stability to an infantile form of walking in which static stable support (Teitelbaum, Schallert, DeRyck, Whishaw, & Golani, 1980) is dominant and must be present for forward shift of body weight to occur?

These observations and measurements suggest that, in devising scales of disintegration of function in Parkinson's disease (Hoehn & Yahr, 1967;

Pedersen, Eriksson, & Oberg, 1991; Webster, 1968), it may be useful to distinguish at least two dimensions of disintegration in gait: (a) coordination of arms with legs and (b) coupling of shift of weight with stepping movements. In terms of separate stages of overall disintegration, it also may be useful for the clinician to distinguish the stage in which swinging the arms during walking is no longer possible without seriously disturbing postural stability. Conversely, in early stages of Parkinson's disease, the principle of indirect amplitude augmentation via allied reflexes may be useful for some patients with Parkinson's disease to improve their own gait. It is also possible that in the early stages of disintegration, systematic training in reautomatization of arm swing might help the patient to regain a more normal gait. It would also be interesting to know whether swinging the arms can be used to trigger walking. Would swinging the arms while standing "frozen" initiate locomotion, or is the role of arm swing limited to the facilitatory modulation of gait once it has been initiated? Such a dissociation between triggering and modulation has been demonstrated in the role of visual stimuli in air-righting in the rat (Pellis, Pellis, Morrissey, & Teitelbaum, 1989).

It should be noted that indirect amplitude modulation via allied reflexes is a principle that operates in normal people also. The data of two normal subjects (one male, one female) have thus far been analyzed quantitatively. When S. B. swung her arms deliberately, she increased 32% in the speed of her gait and 24% in the size of her step. Z. K. increased 26% in speed of walking and 18% in the size of his steps.

Conditions 3 and 4: When S. Y. U. was asked to walk forward heel-to-toe, he did so, quite noticeably more slowly. After a few such steps, he began to sway markedly. When he swayed to the right, for instance, he dropped the ipsilateral arm so that it was closer to his body and raised his contralateral arm further away from his body in a manner that compensated to some degree for the unbalancing tilt of his upper body. This is a normal balancing reaction. However, his arms moved stiffly with some writhing movements of the hands.

Walking heel-to-toe was clearly worse for the parkinsonian patient than ordinary walking. He was unable to maintain his balance and seemed to be trying to do so with his hands, with fingers widespread and moving. It seemed as though he was trying to balance by trying to grab something stable to hold on to, rather than balancing his body as a normal person would, in which case the arms help to maintain the body's equilibrium independently of the external environment.

S. A., the other person with Parkinson's disease who was able to participate in the heel-to-toe walking sequence, did not sway as he walked, so no compensatory arm movements were required by him. Therefore, we have no way of knowing whether he would have demonstrated any balancing reactions if he swayed while walking. We do know, however, that he did not demonstrate compensatory balancing arm movements a year earlier, when tilted suddenly backward while seated in a wheelchair (Teitelbaum, personal observations[3]). It would have been useful to have done such a wheelchair-tilting test also in S. Y. U. because it is possible that he, too, would not have shown any such compensation while seated, though he did while walking. Had S. Y. U. not shown compensation while seated, there would have been more evidence supporting the notion that body support in a person with Parkinson's can exaggeratedly inhibit such compensatory righting reactions of the arms to instability, whereas compensatory reactions may occur while walking. An analogous phenomenon has been demonstrated in the air-righting reactions of haloperidol-treated rats, suggesting that dopamine deficiency reverses the normal dominance of vestibular over tactile-kinesthetic stimuli while reacting to instability (Cordover, Pellis, & Teitelbaum, 1993). This possible shift in modality dominance in reactions to instability deserves further exploration; additional comparisons need to be made to obtain a more complete understanding of the degree of deterioration of balancing in each stage of parkinsonism. Therefore, the earlier observations of Martin (1967)—showing that people with Parkinson's disease do not exhibit compensatory arm movements to sudden tilt while seated—should be supplemented in future studies by an analysis of such reactions to instability while these people are walking.

---

[3]We thank Dr. Silvia Honigman, head of Neurology at Carmel Hospital, Haifa, Israel for helping P. T. to study the arm-balancing reactions to backward tilt in S. A. while he was seated in a wheelchair.

It is interesting that S. Y. U. was much less stable in his postural equilibrium than S. A. was, although his degree of self-initiated reafferent recruitment of reflexes in gait allied to arm swinging seemed better than that of S. A. This suggests that independent submodules of neural function control gait and postural stability (Teitelbaum, 1982) and that Parkinson's disease attacks them separately. It also suggests that drugs aimed separately at the improvement of equilibrium versus locomotion should be developed to enhance the drug treatment of parkinsonism.

Condition 5: S. Y. U. was asked to repeat the activity of condition 4, but with his arms held out at shoulder level to the sides like a person walking on a tightrope at the circus. We had expected that walking this way should help him to maintain his balance: that he would walk forward more easily and quickly, and would do so with less swaying of his body. In fact, the opposite happened: his body swayed much more markedly, almost to the point of falling, and he had to briefly stop walking several times. With the arms held straight out at shoulder level, there is no possibility of using them to hold on to anything. This type of walking requires a pure, abstract, and body-oriented form of balancing. Perhaps there are two forms of balancing: a primitive form that involves using the environment for support to keep from falling, which is characteristic of the normal infant just learning to walk, and the adult form of balancing, in which the arms are used in relation to the body to maintain its equilibrium, independent of external sources of support. It is possible, therefore, that the person with Parkinson's disease can be reduced by the brain damage to a more infantile form of balancing, in which the arms seek external support. This would agree with a previous report that the parkinsonian gait resembles that of normal infants, suggesting that it represents a regression to a more infantile pattern (Forrsberg et al., 1984). The fact that bandage-backfall, a normal infantile reflex, is reinstated by dopamine deficiency in the adult (Teitelbaum, 1977; Teitelbaum, Wolgin, DeRyck, & Marin, 1976) also supports this view. Note also that when supported with its body erect and its feet in contact with the ground, the newborn normal human infant shows a reflexive form of walking that is triggered by tilting its body forward. Such automatic walking continues even over obstacles placed in the infant's way

(Bobath, 1980). Thus, the parkinsonian person may be using such body tilt to trigger an infantile walking pattern, where the gait lags the body tilt.

The initiation of walking by the parkinsonian person is often facilitated as an allied reflex (Teitelbaum et al., 1991) by lines on the ground (Martin, 1967) and by small obstacles (Dunne, Hankey, & Edis, 1987) that presumably elicit visually triggered reflexive stepping over them. It would be interesting to know whether normal infants also show reflexive stepping over lines on the floor and whether this can trigger the initiation of locomotion in them the way it does in adults with parkinsonism. If so, this would further validate the principle of indirect triggering via allied reflexes (Teitelbaum et al., 1991) as a principle of therapeutic value in Parkinson's disease. It would also broaden its implications via the parallel to infancy that appears to link them (Teitelbaum & Pellis, 1992).

Conditions 6 and 7: When S. Y. U. was asked again to walk back and forth across the room and then to do so while reciting the Hebrew alphabet out loud, the rhythmic recital appeared to improve his gait a little; that is, the steps were somewhat larger (an increase of 5.5%), though not appreciably faster. The effect was clearer in S. A.; while reciting the alphabet, his gait was 30% faster and each step was 39% larger. However, when S. Y. U. hesitated during the recital, he halted his walking while he tried to produce the correct next letter. This suggested that two phenomena may have been operating in the control of gait:

1. The rhythmic automatic recital improved the gait. This seemed to be analogous to the counting out loud that is used in the army to improve the automaticity and the synchronization of the marching step of soldiers. Indeed, S. Y. U. told one of the authors that one of the ways he improved his gait by himself was "to walk like a Boy Scout: saying 'one-two, one-two', out loud." After a while, merely thinking it to himself was sufficient to improve his gait and eventually, after a sufficient period of such self-training of re-routinization, he could walk that way without even thinking about it.

2. At a certain point in reciting the alphabet, S. Y. U. appeared to be unable to continue the recitation sequence and, at this point, he

froze for a few seconds, seemingly unable to continue walking. When we listened closely to his recitation while reviewing the videotape, we realized that he had lapsed into a use of the alphabet as numbers, as is done in Israel to label the grades in school[4]. Thus, *aleph, bet, gimel,* and so on signifies not only "A," "B," "C," but first, second, and third grade in school. The subject appeared to have lapsed into this usage as a form of counting because when he reached the tenth letter (*yud*), he followed it not by the letters *kaf* and *lamed,* which would continue the alphabet, but by saying *"yud-aleph"* and *"yud-bet,"* which correspond to eleventh and twelfth grade in high school. At that point, the sequence ends, because there are no more grades in high school. When he could not continue the counting sequence, he interrupted his walking. Thus, if there was a difficulty in sequencing his counting, this difficulty (briefly) prevented him from walking at all. This may reflect a difficulty in doing two things at once, as has been reported to exist in parkinsonism (Caligiuri et al., 1992).

Condition 8: To check further on the possibility of such interference, we asked S. Y. U. to repeat condition 7, but this time to perform the difficult task of counting backward from 100 by sevens. He counted backward, but by ones. We interrupted him and asked him again to count backward by sevens, and started him off by giving the examples 100 and 93. He picked up the sequence at 93, but continued counting by ones. Even when counting backward by ones, the interruptions in his counting were longer and more frequent than those that occurred while reciting the alphabet. Whenever such an interruption in counting occurred, the participant's forward walking was interrupted momentarily. This may be abnormal because although some of the normal persons in our control group had to pause at times when asked to count backward by sevens, they did not interrupt their walking while mentally searching for the right num-

---

[4]We thank Mr. Ehud Katz of Kibbutz Dalia for pointing out to us that the subject was using the first 12 letters of the alphabet as numbers, as a way of counting school grades, rather than as the actual alphabet.

ber. They continued to walk with, at most, a slight slowing in their gait. Note also that S. A., a musician suffering from Parkinson's disease in Merhavia, said that if he listens to complex music, such as Bach, he simply cannot do anything else at all. This phenomenon deserves further analysis.

Although arm swinging hindered I. S., reciting the alphabet still improved the speed and the size of his steps (compare Figures 6A and 6B). Therefore, to improve gait, it can be useful to tailor the behavioral method used by the subject to the degree and type of disintegrations that exist in his walking at that particular stage of his disease.

It should be noted that after completing the condition 8 tasks, S. Y. U. was so fatigued that he had to sit down to rest. This was not so for the normal subjects who performed the same sequence of tasks. This suggests that the degree of concentration required, the actual physical effort involved, or both effects were much greater for S. Y. U. than for normal participants. In a sense, then, the degree of effort involved in the daily routine activities of the person with Parkinson's disease may be analogous to the effort required in the performance of, for example, an athlete. Perhaps the techniques found useful in training athletes to transform complex new motor skills into routine acts (Singer et al., 1994) may be useful for training people with Parkinson's disease to re-routinize their own normal daily acts.

CONCLUSION

It should be pointed out that our observations, preliminary though they are, suggest that the person with Parkinson's disease may be a useful participant in scientific investigations that explore the processes involved in the automatization of motor and conceptual skills (Logan, 1988). A person with Parkinson's disease appears to have lost many of the normal routine sequences in motor acts. Great concentration is required for many of what seem to be the simplest of actions, such as walking. Therefore, the processes involved in such automatization, the losses in them that occur in parkinsonism, and their improvement during re-routinization training should be greatly magnified and more easily differentiated in this disease.

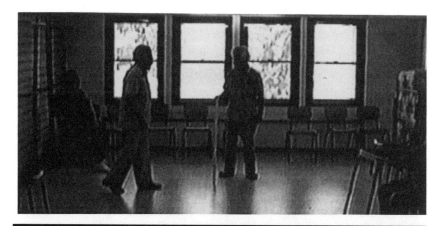

Figure 6 A

Man with Parkinson's disease walking as usual without swinging his arms. Note his slightly forward-leaning erect posture and relatively short steps. (This is the same picture as shown in Figure 3C).

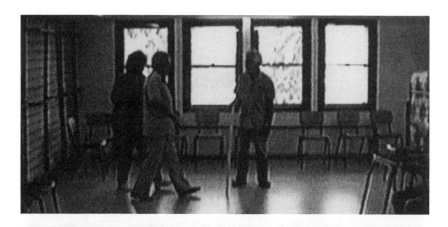

Figure 6 B

Same person as 6A, walking while reciting the alphabet out loud. Note his greatly increased step size and arm swing.

Because of the parallels shown earlier between the gait of autistic children and that of parkinsonian adults (Vilensky et al., 1981), it should be useful to extend the analyses carried out here in Parkinson's disease to children with autism. Thus, we are beginning to reexamine the videotape conversions of the films of children with autism taken by Vilensky et al. (1981). So far, every child with autism has some abnormalities in gait. Most striking is the absence of synchrony between the arms and the legs during forward walking. This can be seen in the position of the arms: (a) in some children, both arms were held flexed at the elbows, about 90 degrees, without swinging (see Figure 1); (b) in some, one arm was extended and swung, while the other was flexed and did not; (c) if both arms were swinging, whether flexed or straight, they were often out of synchrony with the legs. This can be so subtle that the layperson's eye will not perceive it. (Only a written movement notation analysis will reveal it.) Another feature of autism is that the feet and the hands are either ventroflexed (in an exaggerated grasp reflex) or dorsiflexed with the big toe extended upward (in a Babinski-like avoidance reflex) whether in contact with the ground or in the air. The hands are often twisted. When swung forward, sometimes the foot is maintained perpendicular to the lower leg so that the toes are not elevated at the forward extent of the step. This leads to the foot being placed on the ground, not heel first, but rather with full contact of the whole foot at once, as the body bobs downward slightly to accomplish this.

Clearly, as far as gait disturbance is concerned, there are different subgroups among children with autism. But so far, all those whom we have looked at show some abnormalities in gait. Are these correlated with a disturbance in maintaining postural stability and equilibrium while walking, as in Parkinson's disease? Perhaps studying these disturbances in gait when autistic children first begin to walk may be an aid to diagnosis of autism early in development. This merits further detailed analysis.

REFERENCES

Behrman, A., Teitelbaum, P., Cauraugh, J., Moreno, P., Fryman, J., & Teitelbaum, O. B. (1994). When asked to swing their arms, persons with Parkinson's disease walk better with faster, larger steps. Why? *Abstracts of the Society for Neuroscience, 20,* Abstract No. 792.2.

Bobath, K. A. (1980). Neurophysiological basis for the treatment of cerebral palsy. *Clinics in Developmental Medicine No. 75.* Philadelphia: Lippincott.

Caligiuri, M. P., Heindel, W. C., & Lohr, J. B. (1992). Sensorimotor disinhibition in Parkinson's disease: Effects of levodopa. *Annals of Neurology, 31,* 53–58.

Cheng, J.-T., Schallert, T., DeRyck, M., & Teitelbaum, P. (1981). Galloping induced by pontine tegmentum damage in rats: A form of "parkinsonian festination" not blocked by haloperidol. *Proceedings of the National Academy of Sciences, 78,* 3279–3283.

Chesire, R. M., & Teitelbaum, P. (1982). Methysergide releases locomotion without support in lateral hypothalamic akinesia. *Physiology and Behavior, 28,* 335–347.

Cordover, A. J., Pellis, S. M., & Teitelbaum, P. (1993). Haloperidol exaggerates proprioceptive-tactile support reflexes and diminishes vestibular dominance over them. *Behavioural Brain Research, 56,* 197–201.

Creedon, M. P. (1991). Personal communication.

Creedon, M. P. (1992). Personal communication.

Damasio, A. R., & Maurer, R. G. (1978). A neurological model for childhood autism. *Archives of Neurology, 35,* 777–786.

Dunne, J. W., Hankey, G. J., & Edis, R. H. (1987). Parkinsonism: Upturned walking stick as an aid to locomotion. *Archives of Physical Medical Rehabilitation, 68,* 380–381.

Eshkol, N. (1980). *50 Lessons by Dr. Moshe Feldenkrais.* Holon, Israel: Movement Notation Society.

Eshkol, N., & Wachman, A. (1958). *Movement notation.* London: Weidenfeld and Nicolson.

Faber, K. (1978). *Nosography: The evolution of clinical medicine in modern times.* New York: AMS Press. (Original work published 1919)

Forrsberg, H. B., Johnels, B., & Steg, G. (1984). Is parkinsonian gait caused by a regression to an immature walking pattern? *Advances in Neurology, 40,* 375–379.

Golani, I., Wolgin, D. L., & Teitelbaum, P. (1979). A proposed natural geometry of recovery from akinesia in the lateral hypothalamic rat. *Brain Research, 164,* 237–267.

Hoehn, M. M., & Yahr, M. D. (1967). Parkinsonism: Onset, progression, and mortality. *Neurology, 17,* 427–442.

Levitt, D. R., & Teitelbaum, P. (1975). Somnolence, akinesia, and sensory activation of motivated behavior in the lateral hypothalamic syndrome. *Proceedings of the National Academy of Sciences, USA, 72,* 2819–2823.

Logan, G. D. (1988). Automaticity, resources, and memory: Theoretical controversies and practical implications. *Human Factors, 30,* 583–598.

Martin, J. P. (1967). *The basal ganglia and posture.* Philadelphia: Lippincott.

Pedersen, S. W., Eriksson, T., & Oberg, B. (1991). Effects of withdrawal of antiparkinson medication on gait and clinical score in the Parkinson patient. *Acta Neurologica Scandinavica, 84,* 7–13.

Pellis, S. M., Pellis, V. C., Chesire, R. M., Rowland, N., & Teitelbaum, P. (1987). Abnormal gait sequence in the locomotion released by atropine in catecholamine deficient akinetic rats. *Proceedings of the National Academy of Sciences, USA, 84,* 8750–8753.

Pellis, S. M., Pellis, V. C., Morrissey, T. K., & Teitelbaum, P. (1989). Visual modulation of vestibular-triggered air-righting in the rat. *Behavioural Brain Research, 35,* 23–26.

Schallert, T., DeRyck, M., & Teitelbaum, P. (1980). Atropine stereotypy as a behavioral trap: A movement subsystem and EEG analysis. *Journal of Comparative and Physiological Psychology, 94,* 1–24.

Schallert, T., Whishaw, I. Q., Ramirez, V. D., & Teitelbaum, P. (1978). Compulsive, abnormal walking released by anticholinergics in akinetic 6-hydroxydopamine-treated rats. *Science, 199,* 1461–1463.

Segawa, M., & Nomura, Y. (1991). Pathophysiology of human locomotion—Studies on clinical cases. In M. Shimamura, S. Grillner, & V. R. Edgerton (Eds.), *Neurobiological basis of human locomotion* (pp. 317–328). Tokyo: Japan Scientific Societies Press.

Singer, R. N., Cauraugh, J. H., Chen, D., Steinberg, G., Frehlich S., & Wang, L. (1993). Training mental quickness in beginning and intermediate tennis players. *The Sports Psychologist, 8,* 305–318.

Szechtman, H., Eilam, D., Teitelbaum, P., & Golani, I. (1988). A different look at measurement and interpretation of drug-induced stereotyped behavior. *Psychobiology, 16,* 164–173.

Szechtman, H., Ornstein, K., Teitelbaum, P., & Golani, I. (1985). The morphogenesis of stereotyped behavior induced by the dopamine receptor agonist apomorphine in the laboratory rat. *Journal of Neuroscience, 14,* 783–798.

Teitelbaum, P. (1977). The physiological analysis of motivated behavior. In P. G. Zimbardo & F. L. Ruch (Eds.), *Psychology and life* (pp. 2A–F). Glenview, IL: Scott, Foresman.

Teitelbaum, P. (1982). Disconnection and antagonistic interaction of movement subsystems in motivated behavior. In A. R. Morrison & P. Strick (Eds.), *Changing concepts of the nervous system: Proceedings of the First Institute of Neurological Sciences Symposium in Neurobiology* (pp. 467–498). New York: Academic Press.

Teitelbaum, P. (1986). The lateral hypothalamic double disconnection syndrome: A reappraisal and a new theory for recovery of function. In S. H. Hulse & B. F. Green, Jr. (Eds.), *G. Stanley Hall: Essays in honor of 100 years of psychological research in America* (pp. 74–125). Baltimore: Johns Hopkins University Press.

Teitelbaum, P., & Pellis, S. M. (1992). Toward a synthetic physiological psychology. *Psychological Science, 3,* 4–20.

Teitelbaum, P., Pellis, S. M., & DeVietti, T. L. (1990). Disintegration into stereotypy induced by drugs or brain damage: A microdescriptive behavioural analysis. In S. J. Cooper & C. T. Dourish (Eds.), *Neurobiology of behavioural stereotypy* (pp. 169–199). Oxford, England: Oxford University Press.

Teitelbaum, P., Pellis, V. C., & Pellis, S. M. (1991). Can allied reflexes promote the integration of a robot's behavior? In J. A. Meyer & S. W. Wilson (Eds.), *From animals to animals: Simulation of adaptive behavior* (pp. 97–104). Cambridge, MA: MIT Press/Bradford Books.

Teitelbaum, P., Schallert, T., DeRyck, M., Whishaw, I. Q., & Golani, I. (1980). Motor subsystems in motivated behavior. In R. F. Thompson, L. H. Hicks, & V. B. Shvyrkov (Eds.), *Neural mechanisms of goal-directed behavior and learning* (pp. 127–143). New York: Academic Press.

Teitelbaum, P., Wolgin, D. L., DeRyck, M., & Marin, O. S. M. (1976). Bandage-backfall reaction: Occurs in infancy, hypothalamic damage, and catalepsy. *Proceedings of the National Academy of Sciences, USA, 73,* 3311–3314.

Vilensky, J. A., Damasio, A. R., & Maurer, R. G. (1981). Disturbances of motility in patients with autistic behavior: A preliminary analysis. *Archives of Neurology, 38,* 646–649.

Webster, D. D. (1968). Critical analysis of the disability in Parkinson's disease. *Medical Treatment, 5,* 257–282.

Author Index

Subject Index

About the Editors

Robert L. Sprague is a professor with appointments in seven different units at the University of Illinois at Urbana-Champaign. He also serves on the editorial board of *Experimental and Clinical Psychopharmacology*. For the past 30 years, Dr. Sprague and numerous colleagues have conducted research on the effects of psychopharmacological medication, including both neuroleptic and stimulant drugs, with populations of developmentally disabled and attention-deficit/hyperactivity disordered children. His current research involves monitoring the symptoms of tardive dyskinesia, teaching direct-care personnel how to observe these symptoms using CD-ROM technology, and investigating the influences of mentoring in graduate education on the development of ethical beliefs.

Karl M. Newell is a professor of kinesiology at Pennsylvania State University. The focus of Dr. Newell's research program is the coordination, control, and skill of normal and abnormal human movement across the life span, with special focus on the development of skill, variability of movement, mental retardation and motor skills, and the influence of drugs on movement control. Dr. Newell is a former editor of the *Journal of Motor Behavior*.